John Cross Publications

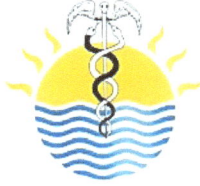

The Holistic Spine - Reflections and Associations
Acupressure and Reflexology in Action

John R. Cross FCSP Dr.Ac.

BOOK ONE

Part One: Anatomy Overview, Spinal Conditions and Their Meaning
Chapters
1. Vertebrae; Discs; Ligaments; Fascia; Arteries; Lymphatics; CSF
2. Central Nervous System; Autonomic Nervous System
3. Spinal Conditions of the Spine and their Meaning

Part Two: Energetic Concepts of the Spine
Chapters
4. Overview of the Subtle Body
5. Meridians and Acupoints
6. The Energetic Spinal Muscles
7. Major Spinal Chakras
8. Spinal Reflections
9. Mental and Emotional Considerations

INTRODUCTION

These two books are my tenth and eleventh publications in a series of books on the practical aspects of complementary therapies that had been planned for several years. The first two discussed acupressure and reflexology combinations in – 'Clinical Applications in Musculo-Skeletal Conditions' – (Butterworth Heinemann - 2000) and 'Acupressure and Reflextherapy in Medical Conditions' – (Butterworth Heinemann – 2001). The third and fourth discussed the chakra energy system - 'Healing with the Chakra Energy System' (North Atlantic Books – 2006) and 'Acupuncture and the Chakra Energy System' – (North Atlantic Books -2008). The fifth was a self-published practical workbook called 'Reflected Energy Pathways – A Practical Workbook for Physical Therapists'- (John Cross Publications -2008) that was subsequently published by Lotus Publishing in 2009. The sixth was 'Concise Book of Acupoints' (Lotus Publishing -2010) that Lotus asked me to write following the untimely death of my colleague Chris Jarmey. The seventh was about my own pioneering type of reflexology of 'Light Touch Reflextherapy' (Author House 2010) that was published due to delegate pressure. The eighth discussed acupressure and homoeopathy combinations in an 'e' book entitled 'Acupressure and Homoeopathy Combinations in the Treatment of Common Ailments' (John Cross Publications 2014). This book was subsequently self-published as a paperback. The ninth was a self-published paperback on 'Distance Analysis and Healing -My Way!' (John Cross Publications – 2016) I have also produced A1 colour posters to compliment the books on the Chakra Energy System, Light Touch Reflextherapy and this one.

Each book has been written for the orthodox and complementary medicine therapist to incorporate touch therapy, energy medicine and healing into mainstream thought. They have been based mostly upon my own personal experiences since qualifying as a chartered physiotherapist in 1970 and registered acupuncturist in 1978 even though quite a few of the theories are built upon the ideas of other complementary medicine pioneers involved in reflexology, craniosacral therapy, polarity therapy and healing. Throughout this series of books, I have attempted to de-mystify the subtle therapy approaches and to show that although scientific and research based medicine obviously has its place, there is room for the complementary therapy approach to healing that is not necessarily based upon scientific research. Much of the work in this book is based upon original thought and pioneering endeavour. It is about energy medicine and is not scientific – I make no apologies for this. My comfort zone is within practical complementary 'hands on' therapies and for me to attempt to discuss my work in modern scientific terms would be alien to me. I find there are two extremes in medical textbooks. Like you, I have read scores of articles and books full of scientific 'gobbledegook' discussing research protocols, double blind trials and placebos for a specific medical condition - that had my head in a spin before the end of the fourth page. Most of these articles (as well as the lectures) I find boring in that there is generally no practical knowledge of how to actually treat sick people!! The other extreme is the one that contains esoteric nonsense that is full of 'head in the clouds' waffle that isn't based upon anything in particular - there may be plenty of practical advice but very little substance. These books on the Holistic Spine represents a 'half way house'. They are based upon my own clinical experiences and findings – that have been taught to hundreds of delegates in practical, experiential seminars throughout the world. Even though they are not scientifically based, and my head is sometimes in the clouds, my feet are always anchored to the ground!

Above all, these books are essentially practical workbooks designed at helping practitioners of all persuasion involved in treating spinal conditions to think 'outside the box'. They will show that anomalies to the spine have significant implications on the wellbeing of the rest of the body. The practitioners who deal with spinal conditions daily, namely physical therapists, osteopaths and chiropractors should be helped with the different dimensions discussed within. Other therapists should learn that the spine and skull have far more significance than just the harbourer of mechanically based conditions. You will be amazed at the number of conditions and symptoms that may be attributable to spinal aetiology.

I became interested in the ramifications of spinal anomalies in my early twenties - having suffered with a congenital roto-scoliosis of the thoracic spine, leading to untold misery for many years and on many levels. Even when I was training as a physiotherapist, answers weren't given as to what was truly occurring with my inner economy. It was only when I became well versed in traditional Chinese and other energy medicine philosophy that the 'penny' dropped regarding many of the symptoms that I had. I shall outline some of these in the text.

Aims of the Books

1. To highlight the significance of the spine and individual vertebrae in the analysis and treatment of visceral and emotional conditions as well as the usual musculo-skeletal ones.
2. To show how the spine may be 'reflected' to other parts of the body and to indicate how these reflexes may be used in both analysis and treatment to complement other approaches.
3. To highlight several aspects of subtle bodywork therapy associated with the spine to give the orthodox and complementary practitioner a more rounded knowledge base.
4. It is NOT intended to be an anatomy and physiology text book, but rather to supplement these by adding practical knowledge based on experience of practice.

Please note that these two books are about the spinal column, but the Occiput and Sphenoid in the cranium will also be discussed as they play a significant role within the practicalities of the Holistic Spine

Part One
Anatomy Overview, Conditions and Their Meaning

Chapter One – Vertebrae; Discs; Ligaments; Fascia; Circulation

One of my favourite books is 'Fearfully and Wonderfully Made' by Brand and Yancey (*Zondervan Publishing House* – 1993). This is essentially a book on religion written by two medical people, purchased during a phase of my life when I was preaching (Methodist Lay Preacher) on a regular basis. Although it may be said that many aspects of our body are remarkable in that they seem to be perfect in shape and form for their given task, it could be argued that the spinal column epitomises this perfection. Yes, I know that tens of thousands of years ago we were swinging through the branches of the trees and our spinal columns were quite different then. I do not accept the premise, though, that Homo Sapiens was never meant to stand and move with an upright posture and that most spinal anomalies occur because of this so called 'weakness'. Spinal anomalies occur through several factors such as congenital and hereditary weakness, accident, injury and wear and tear, and misalignment but *not* because humans weren't meant to walk upright.

Patients are often astonished at the complexity of the human spine, after showing them a plastic model of one. I have always concurred with their awe and amazement but countered it by adding that it is even more complicated than they could ever imagine. I say this in all sincerity because the spinal column not only consists of interlocking bony vertebrae of amazingly complicated shape and form, but it also has the strength to support the body and to protect the central nervous system through carefully positioned muscles and ligaments. When you also consider the amazing 'subtle' body that, in my opinion, is *the* most important aspect, then you have an absolute and utter engineering wonder. If you imagine that our central column *only* harnesses the spinal cord and supports us, you are in for a few surprises. In this book, you will learn that each vertebral level is both independent and *dependent* on other vertebrae for its functions to be fulfilled. You will learn that the spine can govern virtually *everything* – viscera, hormones, energy and emotions.

The spinal column as a whole
As every anatomy student knows the spinal column consists of 24 bony vertebrae -7 cervical, 12 thoracic or dorsal and 5 lumbar together with the sacrum (consisting of 5 fused sections) and the coccyx (consisting of 4 tiny fused sections). Figure 1.1.1 shows classical views of the anterior, posterior and lateral aspects of the spine. Except for the first and second cervical (atlas and axis), there is an intervertebral disc between adjacent vertebral bodies. There are also articular facet joints at each level to allow the spine to move in flexion, extension, side flexion and rotation. The spinal column has three principal functions: -
- To allow movement
- To support the body
- To protect the spinal cord
- Please note how the normal spine in lateral view is meant to have curves. The cervical and lumbar spines are concave posteriorly (lordosis) whilst the thoracic spine is convex posteriorly (kyphosis).

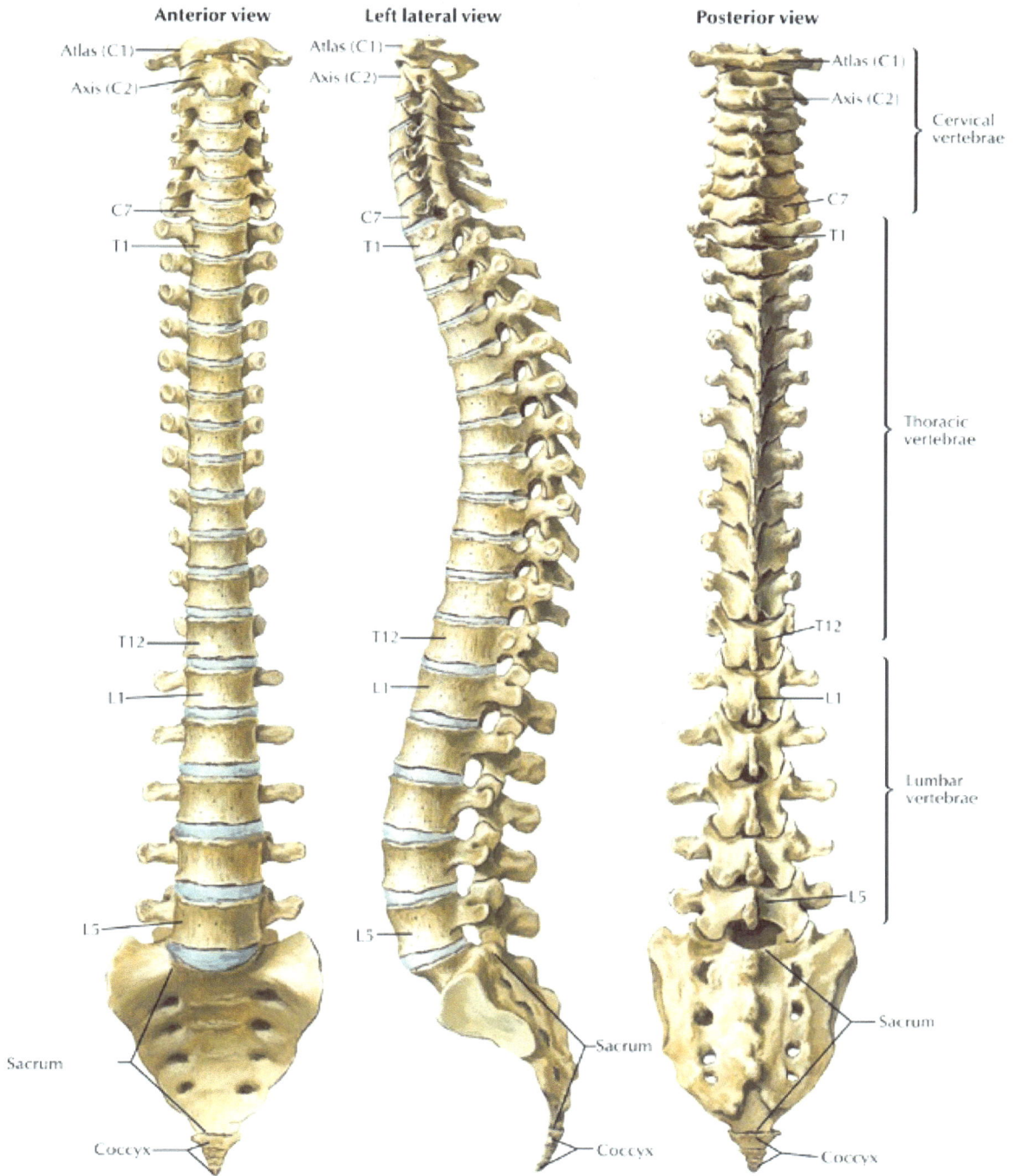

Figure 1.1.1 Anterior, Lateral and Posterior Views of the Spinal Column

When these normal curves change due to chronic faulty posture or disease process, various anomalies can occur to the vertebral level affected together with a reciprocal vertebra. The other type of spinal curve that

5

is not usually normal is a scoliosis, which is a long 'c' or 's' shaped curve in the thoracic or lumbar spine. More about this in later chapters.

Typical vertebra

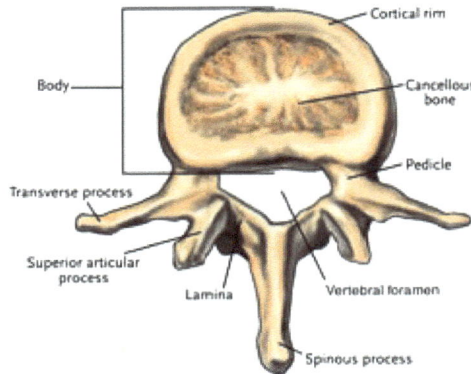

Figure 1.1.2 Typical Vertebra

The typical vertebra shown in Figure 1.1.2 shows the average shape of vertebras cervical 3 to lumbar 5 (C3 to L5). It shows the large circular body which seats the cartilaginous disc, the spinous process that may be palpated quite easily in the mid line and the two transverse processes that may also be palpated but they lie within the outer layers of muscles. The spinal cord is situated within the vertebral foramen.

The spinal complex is composed of different kinds of tissues or systems that may be viewed as purely anatomical or, in the case of this book, as holistic entities that relate to many other parts of the body. The tissues, from the densest to the less dense are Bone, Intervertebral Discs, Supporting Ligaments, Supporting Muscles (in several depths and described in Part Two), the Spinal Cord (which is an extension of the Brain), the Nerve Plexuses, the Autonomic Nervous System, Fascia, Cerebrospinal Fluid, Lymphatic Circulation, Arterial and Venous Blood Supply, Epidermis and Dermis. The more subtle and esoteric systems of Meridians, Acupoints, Chakras, Nadis and Reflexes will be described in Part Two.

Cervical Spine

The cervical spine consists of seven individual vertebrae between the base of the skull and the first thoracic vertebra. They are infinitely small than their lumbar counterparts but, apart from the top two of the atlas and axis are all similar in shape.

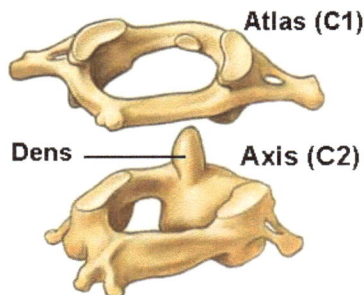

Figure 1.1.3 Atlas and Axis Vertebrae

The **atlas (C1)** is the uppermost (superior) of the seven and is the most atypical bone in all the spinal column. Although it is the smallest with a very irregular shape, it is arguably the most important as it sits directly under the base of the skull. It is unusual in that it is a ring of bone with *no body*.

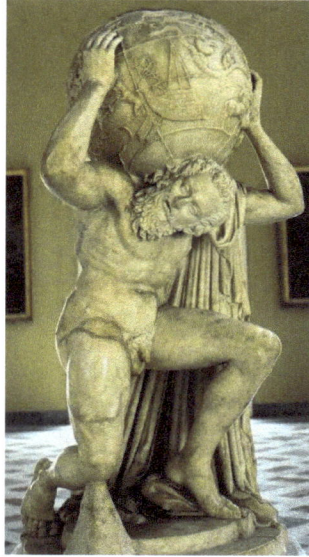

The above photograph emphasises how important this vertebra is! The **axis (C2)** lies underneath (inferior) to the atlas and is arguably the strongest of all the cervical bones. It provides a pivot around which the atlas and head rotate. The dens or odontoid peg articulates with the atlas and is held in place by a very strong ligament. The remaining five cervical vertebrae (C3-C7) are shaped as per the typical vertebra, with the exception that C7 spinous process is much longer – this is the prominence that you can feel at the base of the neck. It also has a single spinous process as opposed to C3-C6 being bifid. The natural curve of the cervical spine is one of concavity. See Figures 1.1.3 and 1.1.4

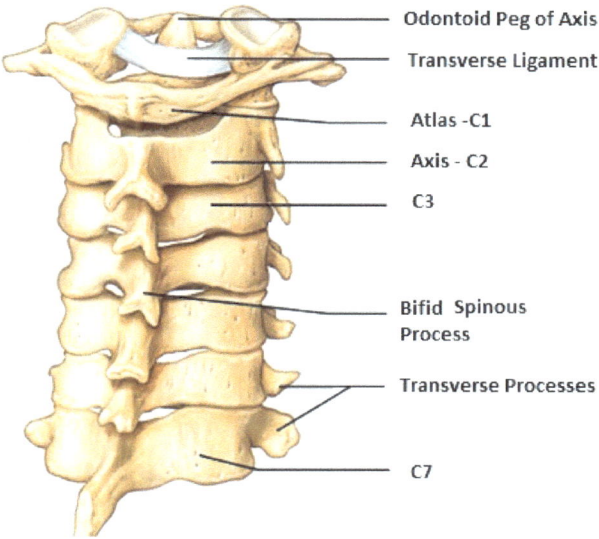

Figure 1.1.4 The Cervical Spine

Thoracic (Dorsal) Spine

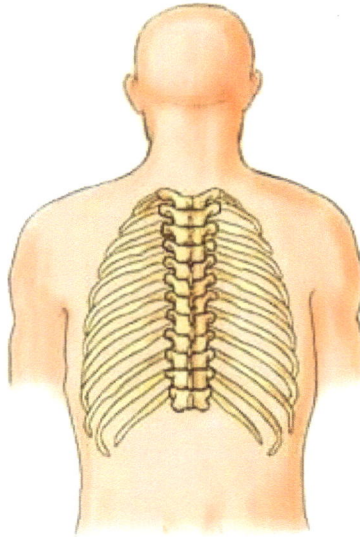

Figure1.1.5 The Thoracic Spine

There are 12 thoracic vertebrae and it is the least mobile region of the spine due to the articulations of the rib cage, that is fixed on the front by the sternum. Figure 1.1.5 shows the posterior view. It is vital to have protection of the heart, lungs and other major organs by the rib cage is that obviously reduces the mobilty. Because of this lack of movement, there are fewer problems associated with this region of the spine. Prolapsed intervertebral discs and other traumatic conditions are much rarer in the thoracic spine, but they do occur. Figure 1.1.6 shows a typical thoracic vertebral shape. Please note the long spinous process and the articular surfaces for the ribs and adjacent vertebrae. The natural curve of the thoracic spine is one of convexity (kyphosis). The thoracic spine is prone to scoliosis of either a 'C' or 'S' shape. This can be a congenital abnormality and vary enormously in severity from very mild (asymptomatic) to severe that often requires surgical intervention. It may also appear during the growth spurt years between 13 and 18 years old and is often called adolescent or idiopathic scoliosis.

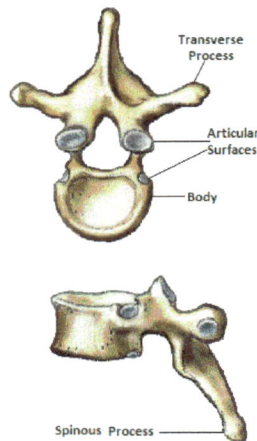

Figure 1.1.6 Typical Thoracic (Dorsal) Vertebra

The thoracic spine may appear to be non-descript and 'boring'. From an energy therapy point of view, however, nothing could be further from the truth. Part Two of the book will give details of this.

Lumbar Spine

There are 5 lumbar vertebrae and they are the largest of the vertebrae that can move via the discs or the facet joints. Figure 1.1.7 shows the anterior aspect and their relationship with the sacrum. Figure 1.1.8 shows the shape of a typical lumbar vertebra. The natural curve of the lumbar spine is one of concavity (lordosis). They are very much larger than the cervical or thoracic vertebrae as they take the weight of the body above the waist. As they take much of the body weight, they are naturally prone to acute injuries and chronic conditions of the vertebrae and discs. The various conditions may result from imbalance with the spine itself, from conditions of internal organs or from emotional aetiology.

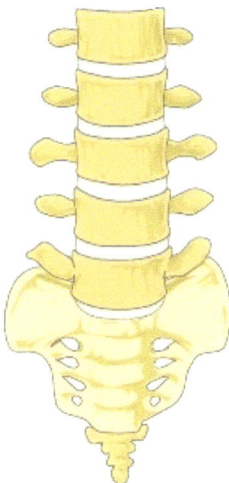

Figure 1.1.7 Lumbar Spine and Sacrum (anterior aspect)

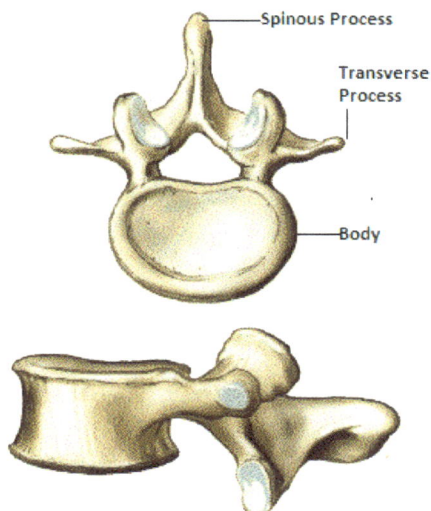

Figure 1.1.8 Typical Lumbar Vertebra

Sacrum, Coccyx and Pelvis

The **Sacrum** consists of 5 fused vertebrae as shown in Figure 1.1.9. It represents the base of the spine and is attached to both the lumbar spine and the pelvis. There is very little movement in the joints between the sacrum and pelvis (sacro-iliac joint). The sacrum is said to be the basement of the building that is the spine and is hugely significant in the study and practice of subtle medicine.

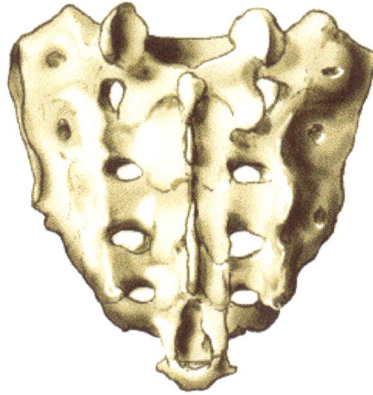

Figure 1.1.9 Sacrum (posterior aspect)

The **Coccyx** is a small vestigial bone, also known as the tail bone. Although it has very little anatomical significance, it is very important in its energetic medicine. It is shown articulating with the sacrum in Figure 1.1.10. This illustration also shows the pelvic ring consisting of the two pelvic bones and sacrum that articulate at the sacro-iliac joint, whilst the two pelvic bones articulate anteriorly at the symphysis pubis. You can also see the acetabulum where the head of the femur articulates. It is very important that this structure remains stable as it is the basement or foundations of the spine. If one or more aspects of the pelvic ring becomes unstable e.g. by a road traffic accident, it presents disruption further up the 'chain' of the spinal column. In energy medicine terms the coccyx is associated with the sphenoid bone and the sacrum with the occiput.

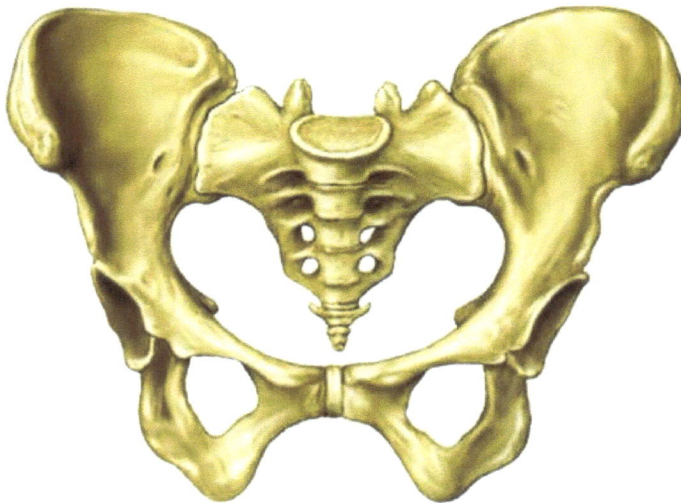

Figure 1.1.10 The Pelvic Ring (anterior aspect)

The Skull (Figure 1.1.11)

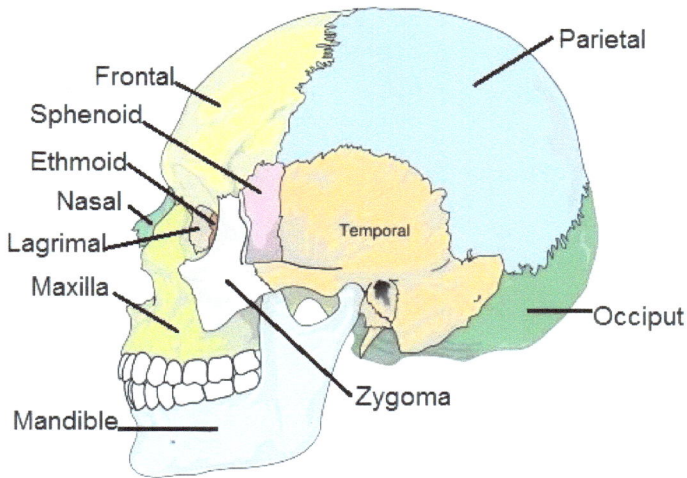

Figure 1.1.11 Lateral aspect view of the Skull

Figure 1.1.11 shows the lateral aspect of the skull with its individual bony parts. The skull has been called 'an awesome looking structure' commonly used to portray death and terror in horror movies. Two bones comprise the skull – the cranium that protects the brain and forms the face, and the mandible. The cranial part of the skull is made up of one each of the Maxilla, Frontal, Parietal, Occiput and Sphenoid and the bilateral bones of Temporal, Nasal, Ethmoid, Zygomatic and Palatine (not in diagram). The two parts of the cranium that we shall describe in this book are the occiput and sphenoid – this is because of their important links and relationships with the spine.

Occiput (Figure 1.1.12)

The Occiput is positioned at the posterior aspect of the skull and articulates with the Parietal and Temporal bones in the skull and with the Atlas at the top of the cervical spine. Please note the large 'hole' in the inferior aspect – called the foramen magnum that enables the spinal cord and meninges to pass through from the brain stem to become the spinal cord in the vertebral column.

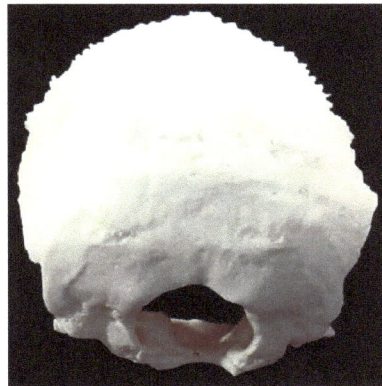

Figure 1.1.12 The Occiput Bone

Sphenoid (Figure 1.1.13)
The Sphenoid is a single bone, although, with practice, it may be felt on each side of the skull at a conjoined region known as the spheno-basilar synchondrosis. It consists of two regions – the greater wing and the lesser wing and resembles the outline of a bat in flight. The centre of this bone -the sellae tursica is important as it houses the pituitary gland. This bone is extremely important in the practice of cranial osteopathy and craniosacral therapy

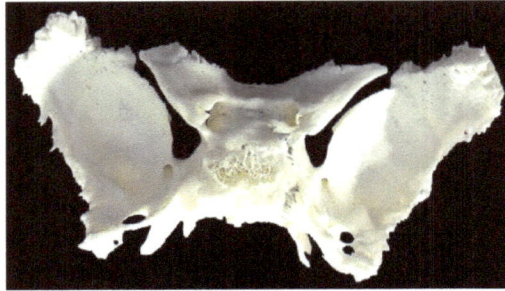

Figure 1.1.13 The Superior aspect of the Sphenoid bone

The bones that comprise the spine and skull are amazingly diverse in shape and size – each, of course, are perfect for their various functions which are to provide support to the body and protect the central nervous system. They are the deepest lying of our physical structures. Bones are living breathing structures and, in energy medicine terms, have the lowest energy vibration of all structures in the body. It is said that the human frame reproduces itself every 7 years and this length of time is essentially the slow reproduction and ageing of the bony system. Other structures reproduce at a much faster rate. Traditional Chinese Medicine (TCM) tells us that bone is supported and governed by kidney and bladder energy.

The Intervertebral Discs

The intervertebral discs (spelt disks in the USA) act as shock absorbers between each of the vertebrae between C2 and S1 and allow a certain amount of movement as well as acting as the main components of load transmission from one vertebral body to the next. There are 24 discs in the human spine made of fibrocartilaginous material. The outside of the disc is made of a strong material called the annulus fibrosus and inside this protective covering is a jelly-like substance known as the nucleus pulposus. As the spine receives pressure, the gel moves inside the annulus fibrosus and redistributes itself to absorb the impact of the pressure. The gel loses moisture as a person ages and the spine is less able to absorb shock. The outer layer of annulus fibrosus on the intervertebral disc deteriorates with age and can begin to tear, causing chronic back pain for some people. Figure 1.1.14 shows the anatomy of the disc. There are several ways that the discs can become problematic and Figure 1.1.15 shows some of these. The disc can degenerate over a period of years by 'wear and tear'. The chemistry of both the annulus fibrosus and the nucleus pulposus changes that often is associated with the vertebral bodies thinning. The disc may bulge, usually in a person who does a great deal of weight bearing and flexion at the same time – such as manual workers. A herniated disc (colloquially, and incorrectly, called a 'slipped' disc) can be the most debilitating of all the disc conditions. The annulus fibrosus tends to get microscopic tears that accumulate to give a tear large enough as to allow the nucleus pulposus to ooze through – thus affecting the spinal cord. The disc may prolapse centrally or laterally. When discs prolapse in the cervical spine this may cause pain along the appropriate root of the brachial plexus and may cause pins and needles (paraesthesia) and numbness in the hand and arm. A disc prolapse in the thoracic spine is quite rare, but does occur.

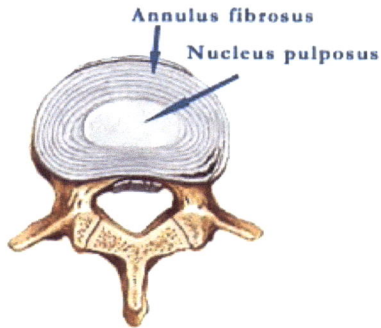

Figure 1.1.14 The Intervertebral Disc

It often happens because of long term scoliosis and vertebral body degeneration. There are no 'motor' nerves that emanate from the mid thoracic spine so the pain and other discomfort is often transferred along the sympathetic chain towards the stomach and solar plexus. Lumbar disc lesions are the most common as, of course, more of our weight is taken by the lumbar spine

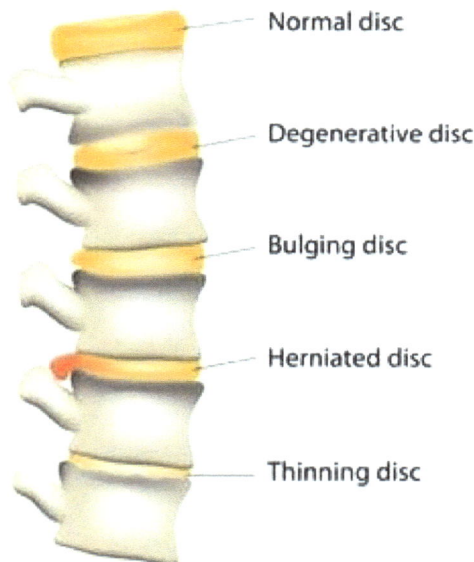

Figure 1.1.15 Types of Intervertebral Disc Conditions

The disc may also thin as in the bottom example. This is often accompanied by osteoporosis or osteoarthritic changes to the vertebral body.

In my experience of treating prolapsed intervertebral discs, over a course of 47 years, it is mostly caused because of sudden movement whilst the brain is switched 'off' and not because of constant pressure. Walking along a street and stopping to pick up a piece of litter gives a classic example of this. If the brain were engaged sufficiently to allow the various muscles that support the spine to switch on, the disc prolapse would be not as common. In energy medicine terms, the discs are associated with the stomach and spleen energies and the lower lumbar ones with the large intestine. Physical anomalies may occur because of internal organic or even emotional imbalance where the symptoms of pain, paraesthesia etc. are merely the final ramifications of underlying pathology that may have been present for many years.

Supporting Ligaments of the Spine (Figure 1.1.16)

Spinal ligaments are bands of tough connective tissue that connect spinal bones together. These pliable bands of tissue permit and limit flexion, extension and motion in the neck and back. They are comprised mostly of collagen. The ligaments hold each vertebra together, and they also connect one vertebra to another along the spinal column. Tendons are similar in structure to spinal ligaments, but tendons connect spinal bones to spinal muscles. The spinal column has a complex system of ligaments that provide a protective layer of tissue for the facet joints and work in conjunction with back and neck muscles to support the spine and hold it upright. The diagram shows the main supporting ligaments that are the Ligamentum Flavum, Interspinus Ligament, Supraspinus Ligament, Anterior Longitudinal Ligament and Posterior Longitudinal Ligament.

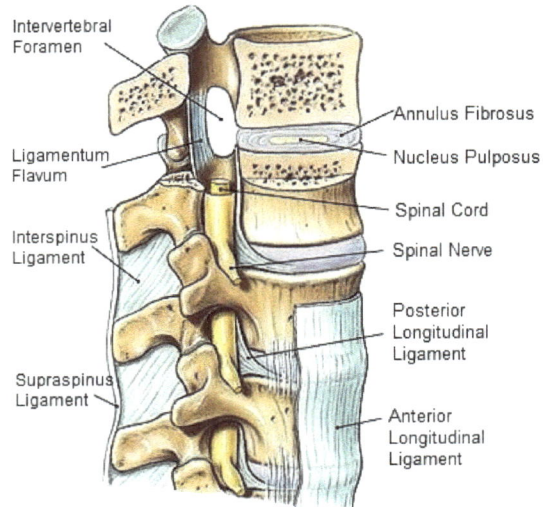

Intervertebral Foramen
Ligamentum Flavum
Interspinus Ligament
Supraspinus Ligament
Annulus Fibrosus
Nucleus Pulposus
Spinal Cord
Spinal Nerve
Posterior Longitudinal Ligament
Anterior Longitudinal Ligament

Figure 1.1.16 Spinal Ligaments

Due to their limited blood supply, ligaments can take a long time to heal when overstretched or torn. Most spinal ligament injuries occur in the lower back, or lumbar region, of the spinal column. That's because we use our lower backs for so many activities and movements, including lifting, standing, running and sitting, among other activities. Ligament sprains are one of the most common causes of lower back pain.

Fascia

Fascia is another type of collagen or connective tissue that consists of 3 parts.

- Superficial fascia that lies directly below the skin. It stores fat and water, allows nerves to run through it and allows muscles to move the skin
- Mid fascia that surrounds and links with muscles, bone, nerves and internal organs
- Deep fascia that sits within the dura of the central nervous system

As fascia is the lining for every internal organ, muscle, bone, spinal cord and large blood vessel, it could be said that it is the one single constant in the human body that binds and conjoins everything. As Thomas Myers writes in his book 'Anatomy Trains' – *Are there 600 muscles in the body or just one muscle in 600 fascial pockets?* So, when we have an injury to, say, the Achilles tendon, it isn't just that tendon that needs to be treated, but it is also important that the links and associated pathways of the tendon, such as

14

circulation, nerve supply and energetic associations need to be addressed to regain the status quo. A modern thought as to the energy flow that we know as meridians is that they are 'housed' within the cellular matrix that we know as fascia. It certainly makes for a fascinating study, and the more we can prove this scientifically, the easier it will be for modern medicine to accept the theories of traditional and naturopathic medicine.

Fascia is, of course, widespread in the spinal complex and it would be impossible to describe it all in this book. However, Figure 1.1.17 shows a cross section of the body at the level of L4, showing the fascial layers and the very important thoraco-lumbar fascia. Figure 1.1.18 shows it in situ. The spinal muscles are given in detail in Part Two and the treatment of spinal fascia conditions is discussed in Book Two

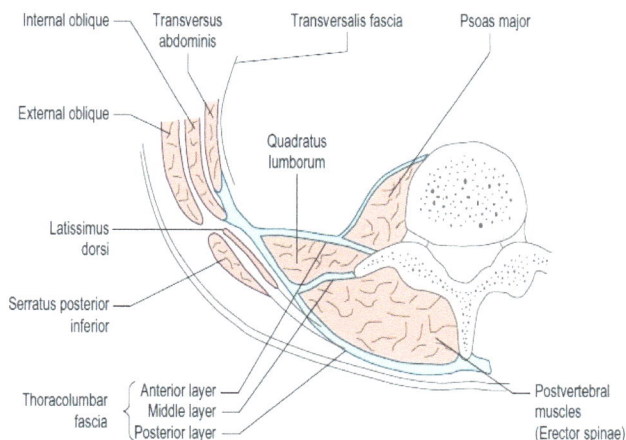

Figure 1.1.17 Cross Section of the Body at L4 showing the layers of the Thoracolumbar Fascia

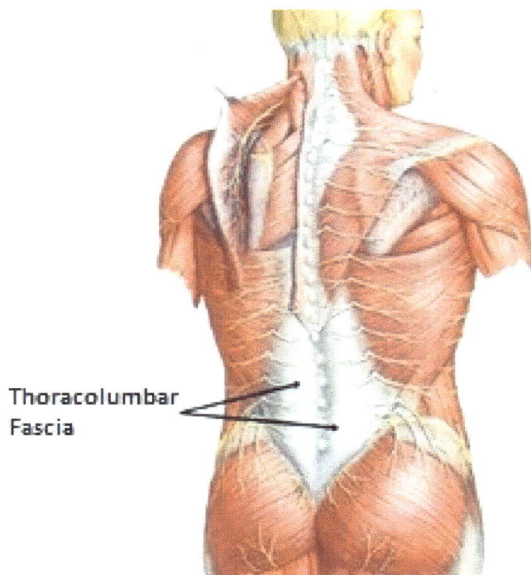

Figure 1.1.18 The Thoracolumbar Fascia

Arterial, Lymphatic and Cerebrospinal Fluid Circulation

The study of the circulation is a vast one so only the essential points are mentioned, that I feel are required in holistic therapeutic practice.

Arteries

The spinal cord is very well served with oxygenated arterial blood and together with the brain consumes over 20% of the available oxygen in the circulating blood. The spinal nerve roots and vertebral bodies are similarly well supplied such as to aid healing of minor, and sometimes major trauma. The artery that needs to be mentioned in detail is the Vertebral Artery.

Vertebral Artery (Figure 1.1.19)

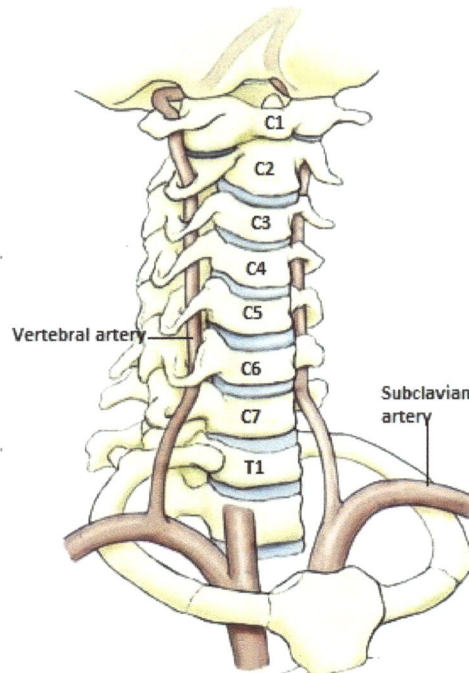

Figure 1.1.19 Part of the Vertebral Artery

Strictly speaking, the vertebral artery has four parts, but it is the 2nd and 3rd part of its course that is of interest to practitioners. It is derived from the much larger subclavian artery and travels upwards passing through the foramen transversarium's of the C6, C5, C4, C3, C2 and C1. As it further ascends it emerges from the atlas foramen medial to the rectus capitis lateralis muscles and curves backwards behind the atlas. It then lies in a groove in the posterior arch of the atlas before entering the spinal canal. As the diagram shows, it has a precarious journey through the cervical region and may be prone to damage. If the wrong type of traction or heavy manipulation is given to the C0-1 or C1-2 facet joints, there is a likelihood that the artery become stretched or ruptured. This could give symptoms of dizziness, nausea or visual disturbance or, more seriously, hemiplegia. It is also prone to stretching around the C6-7 region, where symptoms could be dizziness, and lethargy. The artery may be affected in chronic imbalance such as arthritic changes where osteophyte formation can be challenging. Let me stress though, that in gentle mobilising and manipulation of the cervical spine, and all the techniques shown in Book Two, there should not be an issue with the vertebral artery.

Lymphatics

The lymphatic circulation does not involve the spinal column per se, but the system should be studied as anomalies in the flow can give rise to muscular, fascial and venous imbalance that can affect the viability of vertebral column. The lymphatic system, consisting of channels and nodes, is more extensive than the arterial and venous channels added together. It is a network of tissues and organs that help rid the body of toxins, waste and other unwanted material. The primary function is to transport lymph, a fluid containing infection fighting white blood cells, throughout the body. Lymph is filtered in the nodes which are scattered along the channels. The bone marrow, tonsils, adenoids, spleen and thymus are all part of this system. When spinal muscles become congested, as they often do because of long term faulty eating, poor posture or various mechanical imbalance, this affects the lymphatic flow within and out with the muscle. Thanks to the pioneering work of Dr. Frank Chapman, we can ease congestion by massaging the appropriate Chapman's Reflex.

Chapman's Reflexes Frank Chapman was a doctor of osteopathy in the early part of the 20th century. He found over two hundred regions of the body that felt sore when an internal organ was 'congested'. When these points and areas were massaged, the organic congestion seemed to ease, as if the tension had been removed. His pioneering work was based upon the idea that each of these sore regions was engorged lymphoid tissue within the body's fascia. The areas that are massaged can ease congestion at some considerable distance from the target organ. This is based upon the complexities of the sympathetic nervous system (see next Chapter). I consider Frank Chapman to be a true bodywork pioneer and the profession owes him a debt of gratitude. Chapman's Reflexes are sometimes extremely tender to the touch so they may be used in analysis as well as treatment. The classical approach of Chapman was to give very heavy massage or kneading to the region – without oil on the skin. I would imagine that most of his patients hovered a few inches above the couch, as this, together with Connective Tissue Massage, is among the most painful type of body work that one can perform.

The early days of Applied Kinesiology (AK) in the late 1950's and early 1960's resurrected Chapman's work. The Chapman's Reflexes were coined by the name **Neuromuscular Reflexes (NL)**, and they are still taught as one of the pillars of AK, alongside muscle testing and other forms of work such as acupressure and neurovascular points. The early AK pioneers (see Part Two), instead of using them for organic congestion, dedicated each point to a specific muscle. Most of the body's muscles has a dedicated NL point or area and it is beneficial to give all of them some massage to maintain health. However, if it is apparent that an individual muscle is in a state of imbalance and requires treatment, massage to its NL point will be beneficial in helping the whole muscle. It is still possible to use strong massage on these points and this will be of benefit. However, in the early 1980's I worked out a system that uses both the NL point and a point on the spine that cuts out painful massage when worked together. An interpretation of the posterior aspect of the original Chapman's reflexes is shown in Figure 1.1.20 and the practicalities of my work is described in Book Two.

Cerebrospinal Fluid (CSF)

CSF is produced mainly by a structure called the choroid plexus in the lateral, third and fourth ventricles of the brain. It is a watery, viscous material, similar in chemical composition to lymph or the aqueous humour of the eye. The fluid bathes the brain and circulates the spinal cord.

The main functions of the CSF are as follows: -

1. It protects the brain and spinal cord by 'buffering' these neural structures.
2. It provides buoyancy to the brain, thus reducing pressure at the cranial base
3. It excretes waste products by taking metabolites, drugs and other harmful substances to the blood circulation.
4. It serves to transport hormones to other regions of the brain

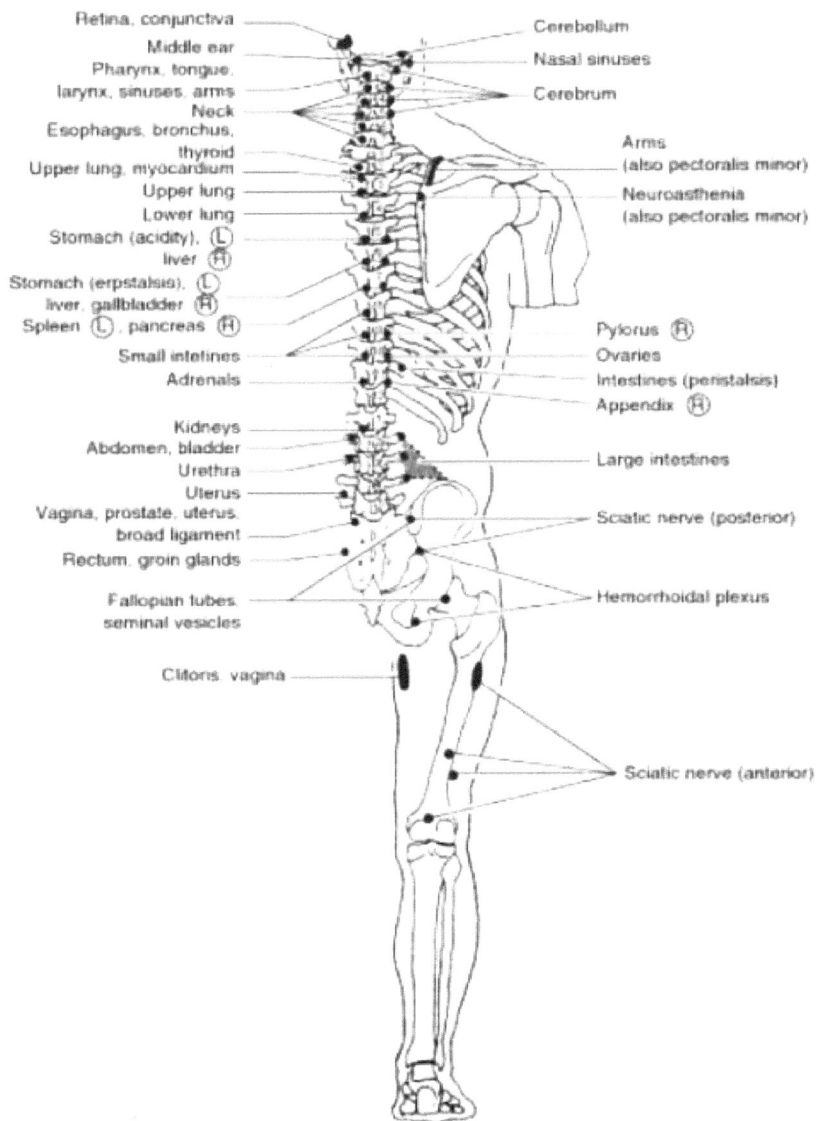

Figure 1.1.20 Original Interpretation of the Posterior aspect of Chapman's Reflexes

The CSF drains out into the blood system via the venous sinuses, maintaining an essential, consistent quality. It is pumped by the 'Primary Respiratory Mechanism' through the Lateral, 3rd and 4th ventricles. Knowledge of the CSF and spinal meninges are very important for those who study and practise Craniosacral Therapy (CST) or Cranial Osteopathy as it is possible to effect dural changes at a distance by holding either the cranial bones or the sacrum. Book Two deals with acupressure and reflexology, but mention will be made on how you can use very simple CST techniques to enhance your treatments.

Chapter Two – The Central and Autonomic Nervous Systems

The Central Nervous System

The nervous system of the body is composed of the central nervous system (CNS) and peripheral nervous system (PNS). The CNS consists of the brain, brain stem and spinal cord whilst the PNS consists of the cranial and spinal peripheral nerves. Figure 1.2.1 shows a lateral aspect of the brain and spinal cord in situ.

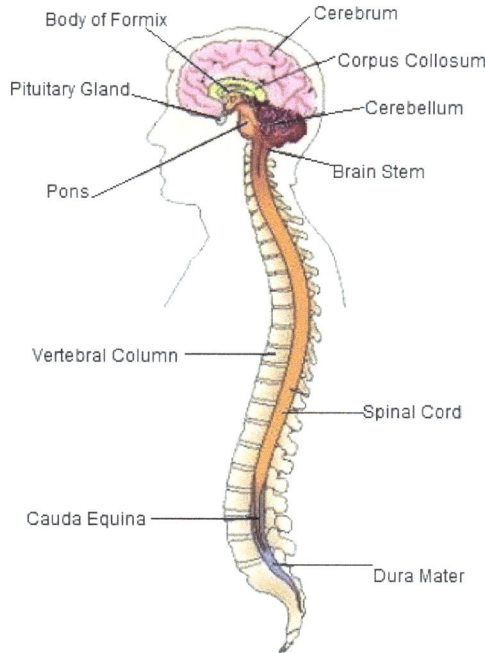

Body of Fornix
Cerebrum
Corpus Collosum
Pituitary Gland
Cerebellum
Brain Stem
Pons
Vertebral Column
Spinal Cord
Cauda Equina
Dura Mater

Figure 1.2.1 The Brain and Spinal Cord (Lateral aspect)

Spinal Cord

The spinal cord is approximately 45 cms. long in the average adult and occupies the upper two-thirds of the vertebral canal, extending from the upper border of the atlas to the first/second lumbar vertebra. Distal to the cord is the Cauda Equina (Conus Medularis) that consists of a system of nerves that descend as far as the coccyx. For most of its length, the spinal cord is cylindrical, but it is enlarged in two places – the lower part of the cervical spine where the nerves that supply the arms are attached to it, and in the lumbar region where it is also enlarged for the nerves that supply the leg. Like the brain it is enclosed with three membranes – the dura mater, arachnoid mater and the pia mater. The dura mater descends below the level of the cord to attach to the coccyx, whilst the arachnoid downwards as far as the sacrum. The subarachnoid space is filled with cerebrospinal fluid. Figure 1.2.2 shows a cross section of the spine showing the cord and the nerves emerging.

The Cranial Nerves

The cranial nerves are twelve pairs of nerves attached to the brain. The origins are from the brain, mid brain, pons and medulla. Some contain motor fibres, some sensory fibres and some both motor and sensory. They are enumerated in Latin (in time honoured tradition) and have many mnemonics to remember them by. Some of these are quite rude, so I wouldn't dream of printing them. They are: -

- I. Olfactory Nerve
- II. Optic Nerve
- III. Oculomotor Nerve
- IV. Trochlear Nerve

- V. Trigeminal Nerve
- VI. Abducens Nerve
- VII. Facial Nerve
- VIII. Auditory Nerve
- IX. Glossopharyngeal Nerve
- X. Vagus Nerve
- XI. Accessory Nerve
- XII. Hypoglossal Nerve

In this book, we are interested in the ones that therapists can affect through the various ways of bodywork, acupressure and reflexology of the spine and parts of the skull. There is much controversy surrounding the ability to effect change in one of the cranial nerves by physical or energy therapy. The following is based purely upon my own work in this field over the past thirty years and contains information that is not discussed in the practical part of Book Two as it is too specialized i.e. outside the realms of subtle bodywork.

- **I. Olfactory Nerve** If the Olfactory nerve has been damaged due to direct trauma or internal pressure, the only way I have found helps in these situations is to perform craniosacral therapy, specifically to the ethmoid, frontal and sphenoid bones. It helps with the flow of cerebrospinal fluid to the damaged nerves. Auricular Acupuncture helps but I have never found it to be long lasting in restoring full nerve function as to re-establishing adequate smell.
- **II. Optic Nerve** I don't believe that any physical therapy can affect the optic nerve, to aid sight. Auriculotherapy has helped with a few patients (using the eye reflex in the pinna of the ear), and the pituitary/eye reflex in the centre of the great toe and thumb also helps, but these two therapies only partially help – certainly not cure in any way.
- **III. IV. VI. Oculomotor, Trochlear, Abducens Nerves** These cranial nerves are the motor supply to the six muscles that work the eye. Once again craniosacral therapy is helpful is aiding recovery if the nerve is inflamed or congested. The occiput is used in this. Although I have not done this myself, some of my physiotherapy colleagues have used specialised exercises to help restore muscular function to the eyeball. Pain in the eye may be helped with acupressure and reflexology – details in Book Two.
- **V. Trigeminal Nerve** The fifth cranial nerve is the most complicated of the twelve. It has a large sensory root and small motor root. It starts life in the pons and travels to the semilunar or trigeminal ganglion, from which it divides into three branches – the Ophthalmic nerve, the Maxillary nerve and the Mandibular nerve. The Ophthalmic supplies the mucous membrane of part of the nose and the frontal and ethmoid sinuses, the maxillary branch supplies the inside of the cheek and the gums of the upper jaw, and the mandibular branch supplies the anterior two thirds of the tongue and the gums of the lower jaw. The motor root of the nerve supplies the muscles of mastication – the masseter, temporalis and lateral pterygoids. Trigeminal neuralgia or migraine caused by inflammation of any part of this nerve can be the most severe of any pain in the body. Although there is no direct neural link to the spinal nerve complex, there is a roundabout link via the superior cervical ganglion and therefore the upper two cervical vertebrae. There is no doubt in my mind that some cases of trigeminal neuralgia may be help with gentle osteopathic or other physical therapy procedures on the cranial base, and C1-2. This is detailed in Book Two.
- **VII. Facial Nerve.** The Facial nerve is the motor nerve to muscles of facial expression and supplies sensory fibres to the tongue, submandibular, sublingual and lacrimal glands. The nerve is often affected as it emerges at the stylomastoid foramen, where it can become inflamed and cause temporary paralysis of one side of the face (Bell's Palsy). This condition is usually self-limiting, but the symptoms may be helped by localised acupuncture (which is excellent) or distal acupressure/reflexology which is covered in Book Two.

- **VIII. Auditory Nerve.** This nerve consists of two branches -the cochlear nerve which is the nerve for hearing, and the vestibular nerve, which is concerned with balance and position in space. The art of chiropractic, founded by D.D. Palmer was developed after he allegedly cured a janitor of deafness by cervical adjustment (see Part Two). Very specialised spinal adjustments called Functional Cranial Release may offer some help in cases of vertigo and deafness. However, as with most conditions (as will be explained in Book Two), if the spine is helped back to full function posturally by freeing the various related vertebrae, it is amazing what conditions may be helped.
- **IX. Glossopharyngeal Nerve.** This nerve emerges from the medulla alongside the Vagus and Accessory nerves. It gives a motor supply to the stylopharyngeus muscle and is sensory to the pharynx, eustachian tube and part of the tongue. It is a parasympathetic nerve as well as being motor and sensory giving its parasympathetic supply to the parotid gland. It may be affected by procedures to the spine and this is covered in Book Two.
- **X. Vagus Nerve.** The vagus nerve is the longest parasympathetic and cranial nerve in the body. It emerges from the medulla of the brain, passes through the jugular foramen, descends the neck within the carotid sheath, passes in to the thoracic cavity, behind the lung, enters the abdomen by passing through the diaphragm with the oesophagus and ends by supplying the digestive tract as far as the descending colon. It is extremely important in therapy, mainly because it is the main parasympathetic nerve supply to the internal organs. It used to be called the pneumogastric nerve, which is very descriptive. It was changed to 'Vagus' as it means 'the wanderer'. It can be affected via the spine in several ways. Please see Book Two
- **XI. Accessory Nerve.** This nerve has two components – the cranial accessory nerve (which joins partly with the vagus nerve) and the spinal accessory nerve which arises in the upper cervical segments, passing through the jugular foramen and neck to give a motor supply to the sternocleidomastoid and trapezius muscles. Spinal therapy will be described in Book Two to treat wry neck and trapezius pain/spasm.
- **XII. Hypoglossal Nerve.** This nerve is the motor supply to the tongue. Its origin is in the medulla. It passes through a canal in the occiput bone to reach the base of the skull to then supply the tongue muscles. Roots of this nerve are also derived from between C1,2 and 3. Practical considerations are to be found in Book Two.

Spinal Nerves

Thirty-one pairs of spinal nerves are attached to the spinal cord, each being composed of anterior and posterior nerve roots, which are attached in front and behind to a segment of the cord, the segments being named and numbered according to the nerve attached to them. The anterior nerve roots transmit motor impulses and the posterior roots sensory impulses. There are eight cervical, twelve thoracic, five lumbar, five sacral and one coccygeal spinal nerves and are numbered C1, C2, C3 etc., T1, T2, T3 etc., L1, L2, L3 etc. and S1, S2, S3 etc. The first cervical nerve root appears between the occiput and atlas. C8 appears below the seventh cervical vertebra and all the others below the vertebra of their name and number. Knowledge of the spinal nerves as they emerge from the cord to supply the motor (muscles) and sensory parts of the body is essential to any therapist who treats spinal conditions.

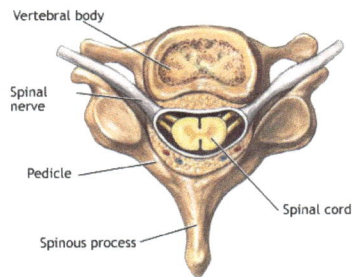

Figure 1.2.2 Cross section of the spine showing the spinal cord

The Nerve Plexuses

The nerve plexuses (yes, it is plexuses – not plexii) are nerves that emanate from the spinal cord that group together to give the nerve supplies to the body. They consist of the cervical plexus, brachial plexus, lumbar plexus and sacral plexus.

The Cervical Plexus

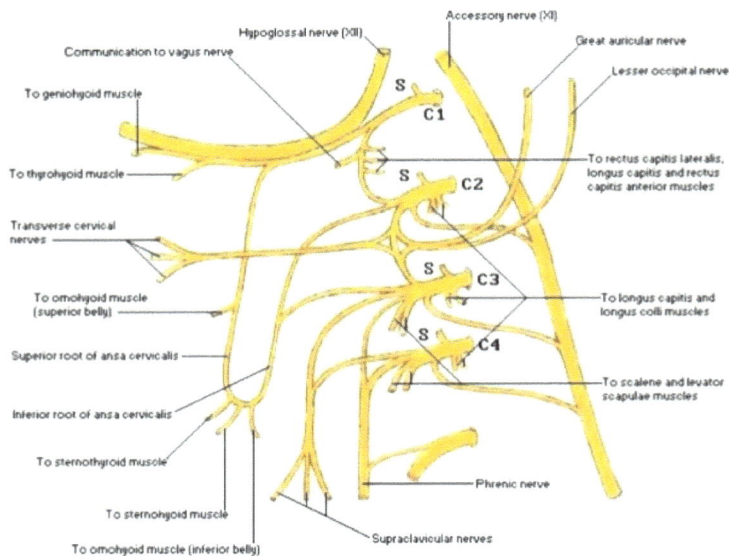

Figure 1.2.3 The Cervical Plexus

There are a few observations of interest to holistic practitioners. Figure 1.2.3 refers

- The Accessory Cranial Nerve XI – this may be affected from the nerve roots of C2-3, C3-4 and C4-5. This is very useful when treating wry neck (spasm of the sternocleidomastoid – SCM) or pain and spasm of the upper fibres of trapezius.
- The Hypoglossal Nerve XII – this may be affected via the nerve root between C0-C1
- The Vagus Nerve X – this may be affected by the upper cervical vertebral roots (see previous section)
- The motor supply to the diaphragm is via the Phrenic Nerve that emanates from between C3,4,5. This is extremely important with spinal cord injuries – any lesion below C4 still has some diaphragm motor innervation. Where there is no spinal cord lesion, any spasm of the diaphragm may be eased with gentle mobilizing and other subtle procedures to the mid cervical vertebrae. An easy

mnemonic to remember the nerve supply of the diaphragm is "C3,4 and 5 keeps the diaphragm alive"

The Brachial Plexus

Every medical, osteopathic, chiropractic and physiotherapy student has the brachial plexus drummed into them sufficiently so that the course of the ulnar nerve – for example, becomes second nature and is often recited whilst sleeping! Figure 1.2.4 refers

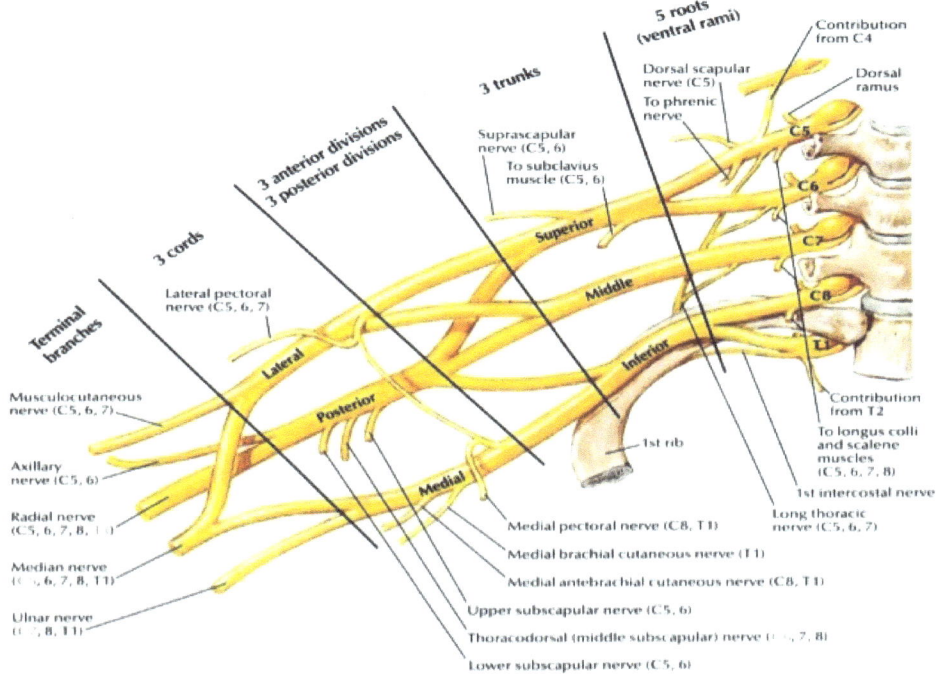

Figure 1.2.4 The Brachial Plexus

I often think of nerve plexuses as railway tracks leaving a station (spinal cord), interweaving and coupling with each other so that pain and other symptoms down a limb may be traced back to its source. If the pain is on the thumb side of the arm, the cause is from the C5-6 root, and if on the little finger side, the cause is from C7-8 root. Please note also how the root C8-T1 (between C7 and T1 vertebrae) overlap the 1st rib. A common cause of paraesthesia (tingling and numbness) down the ulnar border of the forearm is an elevated 1st rib causing pressure on the C8 root (neuropraxia). The main nerves in the brachial plexus are the **Median**, **Radial**, **Ulnar**, **Musculocutaneous** and **Axillary**. The brachial plexus may be affected by disc lesions, arthritis in the cervical spine (cervical spondylosis), muscle spasms and elevated shoulders/trapezius muscles due to stress. Some pectoral chest pains can occur with the lower part of the plexus be affected and can mimic chest pains like ones with some heart problems. This is sometimes called Thoracic Outlet Syndrome

The Thoracic Plexus

The nerves that emanate from between T2 and T11 supply the intercostal muscles that lie in between the ribs. T7-T12 nerves also supply the transverse, oblique and rectus muscles of the abdominal wall. The thoracic nervous system is very important in that it houses the sympathetic nervous system outflow – see next Section and Part Two of this book.

Lumbar Plexus

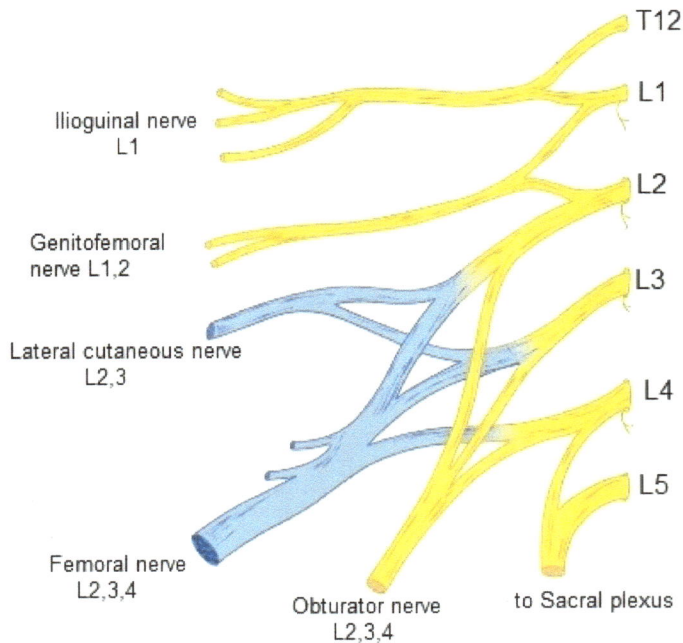

Figure 1.2.5 The Lumbar Plexus

The **Lumbar Plexus** (Figure 1.2.5) is formed within the substance of the psoas major muscle by the anterior branches of T12, L1,2,3 and 4. From it arise several nerves to muscles in the thigh.

1. The **Femoral** Nerve (L2,3,4) passes deep to the inguinal ligament and supplies the Iliacus, Quadriceps and Sartorius muscles.
2. The **Obturator** Nerve (also from L2,3,4) runs through the obturator foramen to supply the Adductor muscles

The **Sacral Plexus** (Figure 1.2.6) is formed from the lower part of L4 plus L5 and S1,2,3 and 4. It supplies nerves to the muscles of the leg and perineum.

The **Sciatic** Nerve (fibres from L4, L5, S1, S2, S3), the largest and longest nerve in the body, passes through the great sciatic foramen into the buttock and then down the back of the thigh into the popliteal fossa (back of knee) where it divides into its terminal branches the medial popliteal (**Tibial**) and lateral popliteal (**Common Peroneal**) nerves. The Sciatic nerve supplies the hamstrings and the two popliteal nerves the muscles below the knee. As well as being the longest nerve in the body, the sciatic nerve is also the thickest, being about 25 mm as it emerges through the buttock (width of the thumb). Similarly, to the brachial plexus, the lumbar/sacral plexus may be affected by disc prolapses and osteoarthritis of the spine as well as a plethora of other conditions and cause that will be discussed later in this chapter.

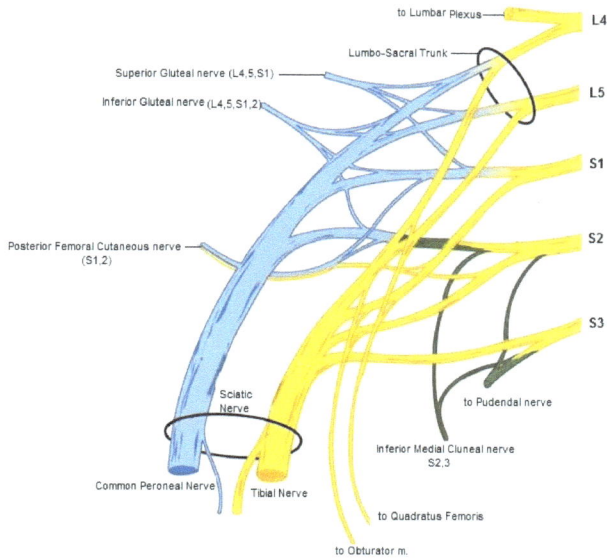

Figure 1.2.6 The Sacral Plexus

The Dermatomes

A dermatome is an area of skin that is supplied by a single spinal nerve. These areas are

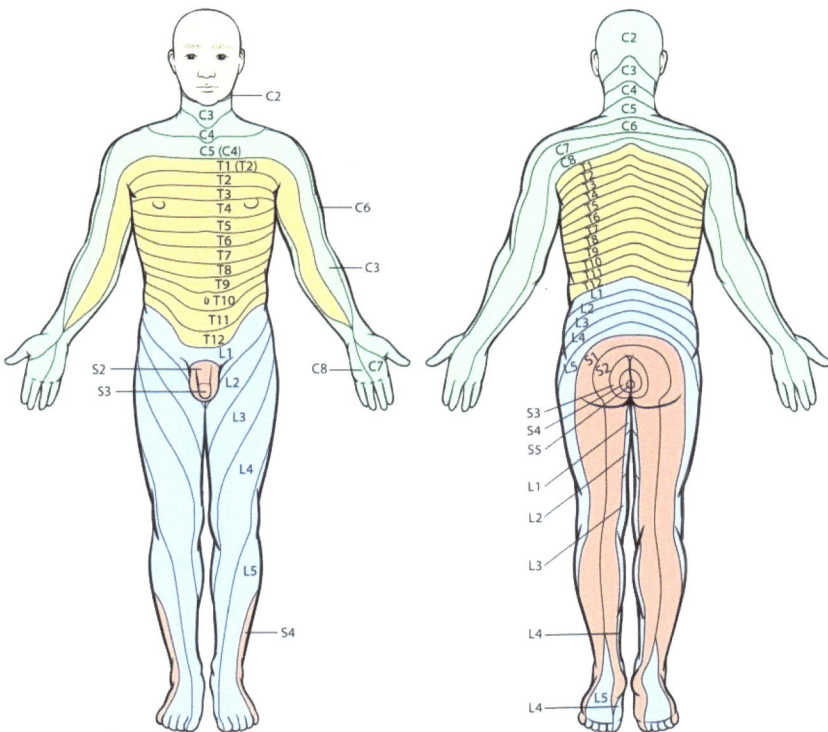

Figure 1.2.7 Dermatomes of the Body

clinically significant in that they indicate which spinal nerve is affected with pain, referred pain and paraesthesia (tingling and numbness) in a region of the body. Please note that C1 does not have a dermatome and the facial skin is covered by cranial nerves. An example could be a prolapsed intervertebral disc of L4-5. This would give numbness in the lower outer quadrant of the leg and the big toe. A lesion here would also affect the tibialis anterior muscle so that dorsi-flexion of the foot would be impaired. The areas shown are diagrammatic as there is usually a considerable overlap depending on the individual person.

The Autonomic Nervous System (ANS)

The autonomic nervous system is part of the peripheral nervous system, but as it is *so* important, it is usually studied separately. Like the rest of the nervous system it is composed of nerve cells and fibres and has both sensory and motor components. The structures it supplies are: -

- The blood vessels
- The internal organs such as the heart, lungs, digestive tract and glands associated with it, the kidneys, ureters and bladder and the genital organs
- Sweat glands, the blood vessels and erector muscles of the skin
- The endocrine glands such as the thyroid, pancreas and adrenal medulla.

It is concerned with such functions as the regulation of the size of the blood vessels. Heart rate, digestive activity, micturition, amount of sugar in the blood and the secretion of hormones.

The autonomic nervous system is composed of two opposing yet complementary parts, the Sympathetic System and the Parasympathetic System. These two systems are different in their anatomical arrangements and in their functions, being usually antagonistic – where one stimulates, the other inhibits. They have been called the Yin/Yang of the nervous system. Both have centres in the spinal cord, medulla and cerebral hemisphere.

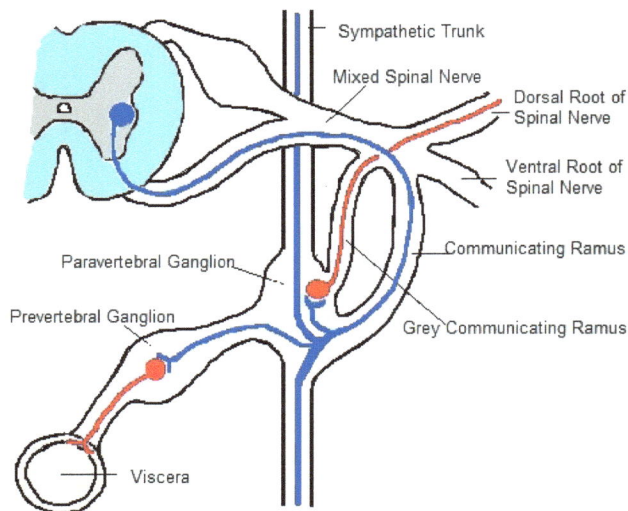

Figure 1.2.8 Diagram of the Spinal Cord and Sympathetic Nerve Trunk

The Sympathetic Nervous System

The sympathetic nervous system (SNS) has its spinal connections in the lateral horn of the grey matter in the thoracic and upper two lumbar vertebrae of the spinal cord. Two chains of nerve fibres, called the sympathetic trunk (or the paravertebral sympathetic chain) run longitudinally on either side of the vertebral column. Figure 1.2.8 shows the spinal cord and the sympathetic nerve trunk. There are 3 ganglia in the cervical spine, 10-12 in the thoracic, 4 in the lumbar and 4-5 in the sacral region, the numbers varying from person to person. From any one segment of the spinal cord fibres may run up or down the chain to end in any one of several ganglia. From the sympathetic chain, fibres are distributed via ganglia to various arteries, nerve plexuses and to internal organs. See Figure 1.2.9 to see this in diagrammatic form. The ganglia vary in size and importance – the largest being the coeliac (or solar) plexus in front of the upper part of the abdominal aorta.

The Parasympathetic Nervous System

The parasympathetic nervous system (PNS), unlike the SNS, emerges from the central nervous system in two separate parts – the cranial outflow and the sacral outflow. Like the SNS it contains both sensory and motor fibres but it differs markedly in that the ganglia are not arranged in a chain but are situated either in or close to the organs they supply. Also, unlike the SNS, the PNS only supplies internal organs and not blood vessels or skin.

The **Cranial** part has central connections in the cerebrum and hypothalamus in the brain. Its fibres arise from various nuclei in the brain stem and leave the brain in the cranial nerves Oculomotor (III), Facial (VII), Glossopharyngeal (IX), Vagus (X) and Accessory (XI) Nerves. These nerves have previously been described as to their accessibility and influence via the spine and the treatment for impairment will be dealt with in Book Two

The **Sacral** part has central connections also in the cerebral cortex and hypothalamus. Its fibres arise in cells in the lateral grey columns of S2, S3 and S4 segments of the spinal cord and run as the pelvic splanchnic nerves to supply the descending colon, rectum, bladder and other pelvic organs.

Actions of the SNS and PNS – 'Yin and Yang'

The Sympathetic system's reactions are directed towards the mobilisation of the body to meet a danger or an emotional crisis. Faced with danger, the body reacts quickly and in ways that fit it best for fighting or running away (fright and flight). Accordingly, the heart beats faster and pumps out more blood. The pupils are dilated and the skeletal muscles get more blood with which to carry out their increased activities. The spleen contracts and drives more blood into the circulation. The bronchi are dilated so more air can enter the lungs. More glucose is provided by the liver from glycogen in its cells for energy production. The bowel and bladder are both constricted. The Parasympathetic system has almost the opposite functions. It provides for a quiet life and conserves energy. It makes the heart beat more slowly and reduces blood pressure. The pupils are contracted and digestion is promoted and elimination allowed. Normal everyday activity is dependent upon these two systems working in harmony.

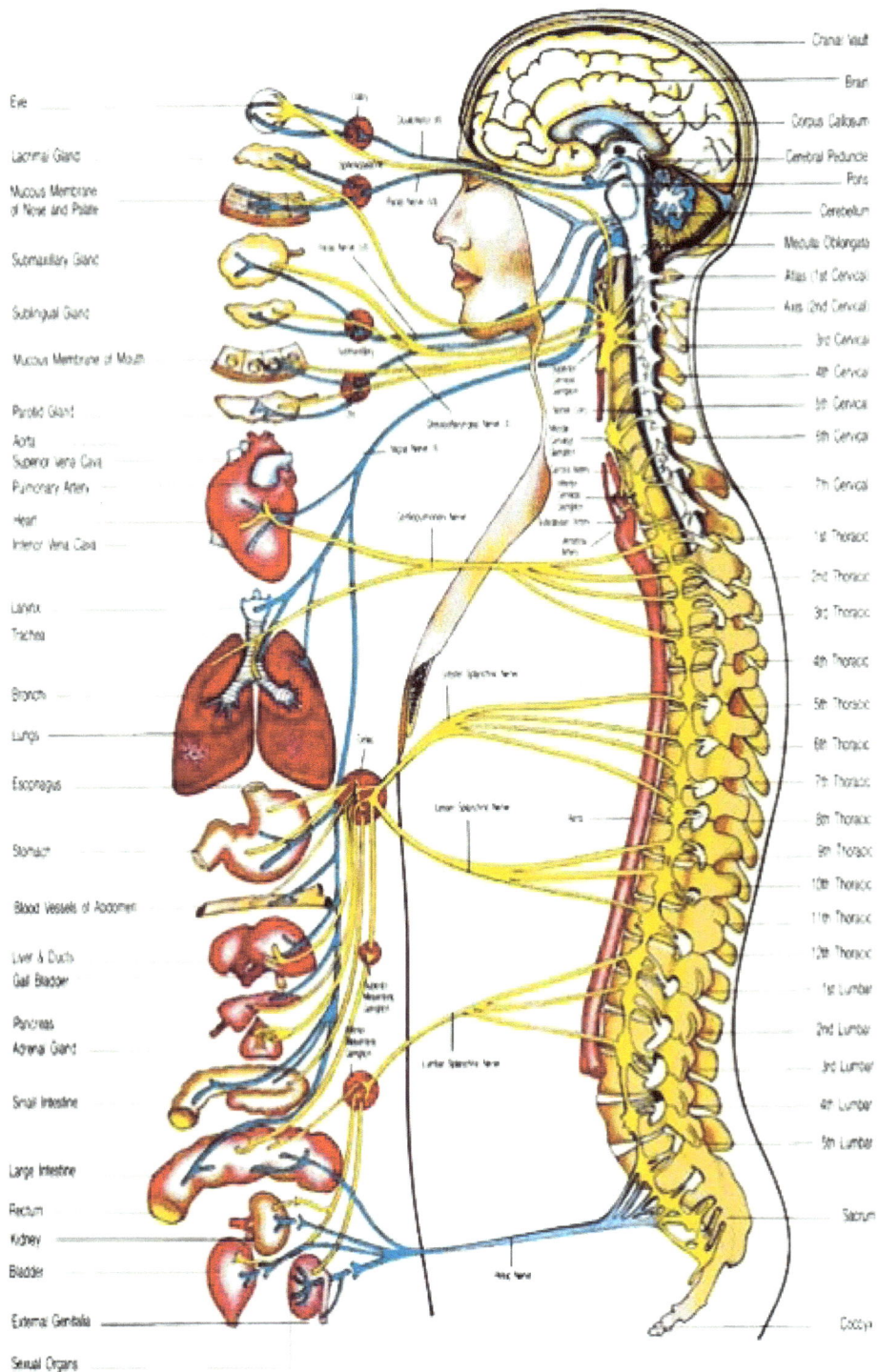

Figure 1.2.9 Diagrammatic Representation of the Autonomic Nervous System

Part Two of this book looks at how the autonomic nervous system is related to spinal energy systems, with emphasis on the Bladder and Governor meridians.

Effects of Spinal Misalignment on the Nervous System

When the vertebral anatomy starts to become imbalanced, for whatever reason, and misalignments and lesions of the individual vertebrae occur, the peripheral nervous system is affected to give us various symptoms dependent upon the level of the lesion. Below is a well-known chiropractic chart that gives a flavour of the region covered by each vertebra and the symptoms that may ensue, in addition to obvious physical ones such as pain or paraesthesia. This chart is used extensively in the chiropractic and osteopathic worlds but may be new for some physical therapists and reflexologists. The autonomic nervous system is involved when the referral is to internal organs.

Effects of Spinal Misalignments

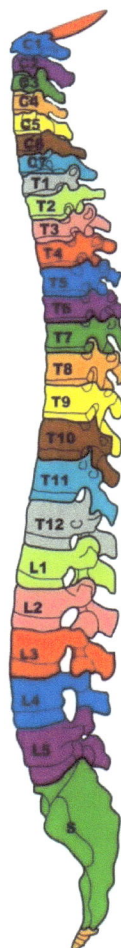

	Areas	Effects
C1	Blood supply to the head, pituitary gland, scalp, facial bones, brain, inner and middle ear, sympathetic nervous system	Headaches, migraine, insomnia, nervousness, head colds, hypertension, some mental conditions, amnesia, nervous breakdown, chronic tiredness, vertigo, dizziness
C2	Eyes, optic nerve, auditory nerve, sinuses, mastoid bones, tongue, forehead	Sinus conditions, allergies, diplopia, deafness, earache, fainting spells
C3	Cheeks, outer ear, facial bones, teeth	Neuralgia, acne, pimples, eczema
C4	Nose, lips, mouth, eustachian tube	Hay fever, catarrh, hard of hearing, adenoids
C5	Vocal chords, neck glands, pharynx	Laryngitis, hoarseness, throat conditions such as chronic soreness and quinsy
C6	Neck muscles, shoulders, tonsils	Stiff neck, pain in the upper arm, tonsillitis, whooping cough, croup
C7	Thyroid gland, shoulder joint, elbows	Bursitis, colds, thyroid conditions
T1	Forearms, hands, wrists, fingers, oesophagus, trachea	Asthma, cough, difficult breathing, pain in lower arms and hands
T2	Heart, including the valves, coronary arteries	Functional heart conditions and certain chest pains
T3	Lungs, bronchial tubes, pleura, breast, chest	Bronchitis, pleurisy, pneumonia, congestion
T4	Gall Bladder and common duct	Gall Bladder conditions, jaundice, shingles
T5	Liver, solar plexus, blood	Liver conditions, fevers, anaemia, poor circulation, arthritis
T6	Stomach	Indigestion, dyspepsia, nervous tummy, heartburn
T7	Pancreas, duodenum	Diabetes, gastritis, ulcers
T8	Spleen, diaphragm	Hiccoughs, lowered resistance, auto-immune conditions
T9	Adrenals	Allergies
T10	Kidneys	Nephritis, hardening of arteries, chronic tiredness
T11	Kidneys, ureters	Skin conditions such as acne, eczema, boils
T12	Small intestines, fallopian tubes, lymph circulation	Rheumatism, bloating, some types of sterility
L1	Large intestine	Constipation, colitis, diarrhoea, hernias
L2	Appendix, upper leg, caecum	Appendicitis, cramps, acidosis, varicosities
L3	Sex organs, ovaries or testicles, uterus, bladder, knee	Cystitis and bladder stricture, painful periods, bed wetting, impotency, menapausal symptoms
L4	Prostate gland, lower spinal muscles, sciatic nerve	Sciatica, lumbago, backache, dismennorrhia, frequent urination
L5	Lower legs, ankles, feet, toes	Poor circulation, varicosities, swollen ankles, weak ankles, leg cramp
Sacrum	Hip joints and buttocks	Sacro-iliac conditions, lordosis and other spinal curvatures
Coccyx	Rectum, anus	Haemorrhoids, pruritis, coccydinia

Figure 1.2.10 Areas and Effects of Spinal Misalignments

Please note that this chart covers how vertebral lesions affect the peripheral nervous system. It is *not* a chart that covers the *energy* flow at each level. In my naturopathic student days, I spent many a sleepless night trying to correlate this chart with the ones that discuss the inner and outer bladder meridian lines and the symptoms that they give when affected- they are not the same and do not correlate with each other. The meridian system is discussed in Part Two of this book and the overall symptoms that ensue at each vertebral level are given in Book Two.

Are the Spinal Nerves straightforward?
So far, mention has been made of cranial nerves, spinal nerves (composing of motor and sensory) and the autonomic nerves (composing of sympathetic and parasympathetic). We have already seen that some cranial nerves may be motor, sensory or parasympathetic. So, is it possible that the rigid anatomical nervous system (that I learnt fifty years ago) may have some surprises and not what it seems? The latest research shows that some sympathetic nerves may act as both sensory and motor and that the cranial parasympathetic nerves may reverse their role to become sympathetic given the right situations. Although pain is a complicated subject and multifactorial, it is assumed that pain stems from the sensory nerves that emit from the spinal cord. It has now been shown that visceral pain may occur when the sympathetic ganglion is affected (by direct trauma or stress) – [The Physiotherapy Pain Association - *Topical Issues in Pain 3* – Louis Gifford (Ed)], CNS Press 2002. Naturopaths and ye olde osteopaths have always known that they are able to ease visceral pain through easing 'trapped nerves' in the spine, but scientific research has now shown this to be a fact. An example of this would be an imbalance in the mid thoracic spine caused by scoliosis, arthritic changes or trauma may give pain to the stomach or oesophagus, causing the stomach to become hypersensitive to foods etc. that hitherto were tolerated. I also believe that when the vagus nerve is affected, again by trauma or stress, it can act sympathetically and *cause* the overloading of neural tension that it usually prevents. If one can avoid stress and positively engage in stress busting exercises such as meditation, yoga, physical activity etc. this will enhance the parasympathetic system to prevent overload on the sympathetic system even though there may be spinal issues. These thoughts will be expanded in Book Two in a section on self-healing.

Case History 1

Male (LKD)– mid 60's – complained of stomach pain only when he did exercise or even walked longer than 100 metres. When the exercise ceased, the stomach pain eased. Before I saw him, he'd received ultra sound scan, endoscopy and a balloon endoscopy, plus several different drugs all aimed at easing the 'obvious' indigestion symptoms (albeit unusual) that the medical profession thought he had. Each test proved negative, except during the first endoscopy, the pain that he felt was elicited the moment that the probe travelled through the cardiac sphincter. He was discharged by the abdominal surgery team as 'probably cardiac or emotional' When I saw him, I examined his spine. He had chronic cervical spondylosis and he also told me that he had a 'slipped' L4-5 disc. He also told me that he had a history of diaphragmatic tension, anxiety, mild indigestion and arrhythmia. I suggested he had an MRI of the mid thoracic spine. (In the UK, only a medical consultant can order an MRI if done on the national health service (NHS), but I could refer him if he had it carried out privately – this he did. He returned with both CD rom film and report. It showed that there was a disc prolapse of T6-T7. He was taught specific exercises to strengthen the thoracic muscles and given acupuncture locally to the mid thoracic spine as well as to the lower cervical and lower lumbar spine. The pain started to ease after three sessions and if he exercises correctly, it does not return.

This patient highlights the fact that some visceral pain is caused by spinal nerve tension. The fact that he had a mid-thoracic disc prolapse (quite rare) was the obvious cause of his pain. We take it for granted that pain and inflammation of the lower cervical region will give referred pain in the brachial plexus down the arm, and that referred pain from the lumbo-sacral region will affect the lower limb. What happens to pain from a mid-thoracic source – it must go somewhere!! What happens is that it causes the cardiac sphincter (between the oesophagus and stomach) to go into spasm, and spasm creates pain. Sadly, I have yet to meet a single abdominal specialist who will admit that some abdominal symptoms are referred from the spine. It isn't yet part of the orthodox canon.

Chapter Three – Spinal Conditions and their Meaning

 You may think that a sprain is caused by forced movement of the joint, that a strain is caused by a muscle suddenly going 'tight' and that a 'slipped' disc just "happens". Many seemingly accidental lesions of the mechanical body have their aetiology in non-mechanical territory. There are many excellent books available about mind-body relationships, explaining how our emotions may cause imbalance within the structure of the whole body. In this book, I discuss the many mind-body factors affecting the spine, that has not been covered, at least not in depth, in any other book I have seen. Below is, what I consider, to be the most important illustration in the book. Figure 1.3.1 shows the classical healing triad, that also serves as the assessment or diagnostic triad.

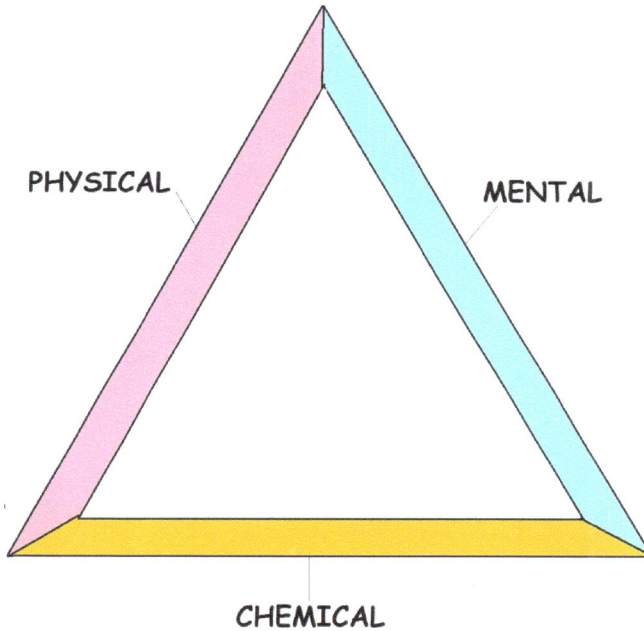

PHYSICAL

MENTAL

CHEMICAL

Figure 1.3.1 The Healing Triad

Natural medicine (naturopathy) recognises that disease may be due to inherited, congenital or developmental factors as well as infection, trauma, nutritional, structural and emotional imbalances. It recognises that the human body is made up of physical, chemical and mental attributes, collectively known as the healing triad and that there is an amazing interaction between these three bodily systems. When you meet the patient for the first time and start to build up the Case Sheet, the history of chemical and emotional imbalance is just as important as the structural history of accidents and injuries.

Physical The physical aspect of the spine consists of the skull and vertebrae, supporting muscles, ligaments, fascia and nervous system

Chemical The chemical influence upon the spine would come from food, liquids and toxins that are ingested via the mouth, lungs or skin. The hormones that are secreted via the endocrine glands, blood, lymph and cerebrospinal fluid also come into this category.

Mental (Emotional) The mental aspects that may influence the spine come from our thoughts, habits, behaviour, the type of 'character' we are, our 'spirituality and personality', our reactions to external influences that affect our lives such as fear, grief, sadness or guilt. This Part of the book will deal with the spinal tissues and how they can be influenced by chemical and mental imbalances. The final chapter of Part 2 will deal with the 'character and personality' of a person and how they influence each level of the spine.

You will all have heard of the, now rather hackneyed, phrase of 'You are what you eat'. This is undoubtedly true. If you eat rubbish, you will become rubbish in body and mind. There is little doubt that what we eat affects the maintenance of health and helps improves dis-ease factors. I believe, though, that a greater truism is 'You become what you think'. Constant negativity, anxiety, depression, fear or other external forces that are beyond our coping facilities affect the body in general, and the spine is no exception in this. I shall cover how the chemical (food, liquids etc.) and emotional (anger, grief etc.) affect the physical structure of the spine.

Aetiology of Spinal Imbalance
There are three different root causes of imbalance to the spine – physical, chemical and emotional. These often don't appear in isolation as they are so intrinsically bound together. An obvious physical cause of imbalance e.g. accident or injury may eventually bring about chemical and emotional imbalance, that, in turn makes the original condition worse. We have beautifully constructed spines that start to become less than perfect only when we do something to alter the status quo – in other words, it is virtually always our own fault for any kind of spinal anomaly. The obvious exception to this is when we are born with a spinal deformity either of a congenital nature or an herediteral imbalance. Let me state clearly that wear and tear conditions of the spine do not occur due to being overweight or because we exercise too much. The most common way that spines start to become less than perfect is due to *misalignment*. This may result from an accident or injury, causing the spinal supporting muscles to go into spasm and overstretching of the spinous ligaments. This, in turn will cause localised inflammation and misalignment that will affect the facet joints of ligaments. Then because we always need to keep our eyes level, the postural imbalance of the lesion site is soon referred to another region of the spine as a compensatory effect. Many examples of this are in later chapters.

Physical Causes of Spinal Conditions
An excellent synopsis of this is given by Sarah Key in her book 'The Back-Sufferer's Bible' (Random House – 2000). She states that a simple back pain develops when an intervertebral disc loses water content and stiffens. This could be caused by compression or poor posture. She then postulates that if untreated in the acute phase, other stages of decrepitude would ensue, namely – a stiff spinal segment, arthritic changes of the facet joints, an acute locked back, a prolapsed (slipped) intervertebral disc and, finally, an unstable segment. The aetiology and treatment of these states of spinal anomaly can be found, not only in Sarah Key's book but in hundreds of others dedicated to osteopaths, chiropractors or physical therapists. Because this book is concerned with holism and looking 'outside the box', we shall not dwell any longer on physical causes.

Chemical Causes of Spinal Conditions

Water – Referring to the previous paragraph where Sarah Key suggests that back pain is initiated when the intervertebral disc starts to lose water content, this gives an enormous clue as to how to prevent, not only spinal anomalies, but also general imbalance in the body's connective tissue. Adequate hydration is essential for good health, especially ligaments, fascia and synovial joints. I have lost count the number of patients to whom I have given the simple advice of drinking more water to reduce joint stiffness. It is such an *easy* thing to do, but one that people do not seem to be aware of. It is also essential that the fluid intake is *water* – not tea or coffee, and certainly not sugary drinks.
Sugar – We all recognise the perils of eating foods containing too much sucrose in that it is one of the main causes of overweight, diabetes, cancers and many other conditions. One of the main reasons why sucrose is so detrimental is that it is a complicated chained molecule – C17 H36 O18. This produces a great deal of acid in the system – or rather the stomach produces hydrochloric acid to break this food down to a simpler

carbohydrate. The excess acid goes to the person's weakness, the joints and connective tissues. People who eat natural foods, preferably raw food, have fewer spinal conditions.

Red meat - Eating too much red meat, once again produces excess acid in the digestive system. This tends to affect the lumbar supporting muscles such as the erector spinae. A common cause of fibromyalgia is the over consumption of red meat.

Refined carbohydrates – over indulgence in refined carbohydrates over a long period of time will cause weakened abdominal muscles, that, in turn, causes lumbar lordosis and chronic lumbar spine imbalance.

Mental (Emotional) Causes of Spinal Conditions

To adequately describe this complicated issue, we shall begin with some traditional philosophy: -

The Law of Five Transformations (Elements)

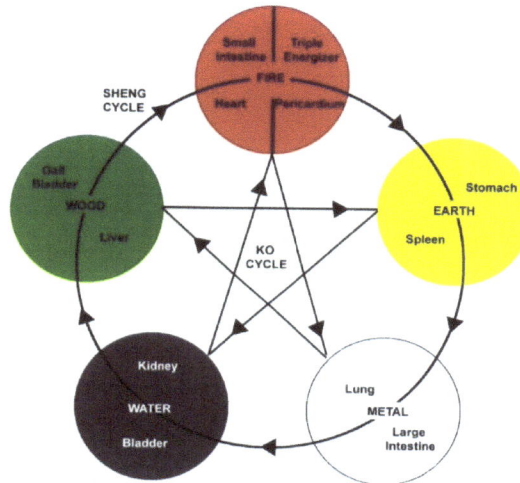

	FIRE	EARTH	METAL	WATER	WOOD
Direction:-	South	-	West	North	East
Colour:-	Red	Yellow	White	Black	Green
System:-	Circulation	Connective	Skin	Bones	Muscles
Face:-	Mouth	Tongue	Nose	Ears	Eyes
Emotion:-	Joy	Sympathy	Grief	Fear	Anger
Season:-	Summer	Late Summer	Autumn	Winter	Spring
Weather:-	Heat	Humidity	Dryness	Cold	Wind
Taste:-	Bitter	Sweet	Pungent	Putrid	Sour

Figure 1.3.2 The Law of Five Transformations (Elements)

The above diagram, beloved of traditional Chinese medicine practitioners and students, shows the five Elements of Fire, Earth, Metal, Water and Wood and how they interact with each other and with the human body. Please note that these Elements (upper case 'E' purposely written) may differ to the Elements described by other traditional philosophies and the more modern ones, including Polarity Therapy. This Law has huge ramifications and is extremely important when diagnosing and treating using traditional acupuncture/acupressure. All aspects of this fascinating Law are important, but it is the Systems and Emotions that will be discussed here. Each of the Elements represents two or four internal organs, that, in turn, are said to energetically control various systems and emotions. The movement of energy from organ to organ is important, not only in treatment, but also in analysing the state of the body and predicting outcomes if treatment was not given (more of this later in the chapter)

Water Element – This Element consists of the **Kidney** (yin) and **Bladder** (yang) organs. It is said to influence **Bone**. The skeleton represents the deepest of the physical tissues, and in energetic terms, the least vibrant and slowest growing. When these two organs are in a state of imbalance or dis-ease, this can affect the strength of the bony structures. It is no accident that the traditional Oriental medicine of acupuncture places the kidney energy channel (meridian) vertically either side of the anterior mid line and the bladder channel vertically either side of the spine. These are explained in detail in Part Two. Furthermore, the kidney channel terminates around the anterior aspect of the throat at the medial aspect of the clavicle and energises the parathyroid glands at this level of the body. [The parathyroid glands are important in affecting the growth and repair of bone tissue]. The Water Element is also in charge of the central and autonomic nervous systems. The emotional aspects of Kidney and Bladder energies are **Fear**, **Anxiety** and some **Phobias**. Fear, of course, is the primal sensation in many emotional conditions and dis-eases. The kidneys are the root of life, and our energies and will to succeed in life are rooted in healthy kidney energy. Poor kidney function leads to general malaise and the inability to face the rigours of life. The kidney energetic system is also the main 'ancestral energy' i.e. the amount of energy with which we are born, including our constitution. This is mainly dependent on our parent's vital force and our conditions during gestation and birth. Although kidney and bladder energies deal with the whole of the spinal column, they are specifically dominant in the lumbo-sacral region. So, a strong water Element will lead to a strong lower spine. In ayurvedic therapy, the kidney energy is related to the Base chakra (located at the coccyx).

Wood Element – This Element consists of the **Liver** (yin) and **Gall Bladder** (yang) organs. It is said to influence **Muscles and Tendons.** The Liver influences muscular tissue and the Gall Bladder influences tendons. I appreciate that this conclusion is different to many other interpretations that consider the Spleen to influence muscles. However, this is what I learnt 40 years ago at acupuncture college, and my mind has not been swayed away from this 'fact', because in practical terms, and dealing with sick people, it is borne out time and time again. So, when either the Liver or Gall Bladder energetic systems are in a state of imbalance, the musculature and tendons of the body are affected, including the spine. The emotional aspects of the Wood Element are **Anger, Irritability, Resentment, Frustration and Irrational Behaviour.** Poor liver or gall bladder function can lead to these emotional traits or be caused by them (it is a two-way operation). Stress of any aetiology will always affect the liver and put strain on the spinal muscles – especially the ones that support the lower cervical and mid thoracic spine. As you will read in Part Two, Applied Kinesiology philosophy gives the twelve meridians (and their internal organic counterparts) related to each different muscle – but that is a different energetic concept.

Fire Element – This Element consists of the **Heart** (yin), **Small Intestine** (yang) and **Pericardium** (yin) plus the non-organ of the **Triple Energizer** (yang) and is the only Element that contains more than two individual parts. The Heart influences blood circulation and, as such, is closest to the orthodox way of viewing medicine. The Pericardium is closely allied to the Heart and is seen as the Heart Protector. Old terminology calls this organ/meridian the Heart Constrictor. The newer term for the Pericardium in Applied Kinesiology is 'Circulation-Sex' – which I loathe and detest! Both the Heart and Pericardium deals with **Joy and Love**. Both, of course, are positive emotions and whilst they are positive there is little pathology with the organs or circulation. However, when joy is missing (hate or sadness), this can, and does affect both the Heart energy and free flowing circulation. The Small Intestine is involved with separating the pure from the impure. Its emotional counterpart is **Assimilation**. The Triple Energizer or San Jiao is a complicated traditional concept and regulates water and other fluids in three aspects of the body – traditionally called heaven, earth and man. This energetic concept is to do with our spiritual aspect (or Shin), and works alongside the Heart in this.

Earth Element – This Element consists of the **Spleen** (yin) and **Stomach** (yang) organs. The Spleen's functions in traditional Oriental medicine differ from the orthodox way of looking at the spleen. It is the main organ of digestion as well as lymphatic flow. The main tissues governed by Spleen energy are **Connective Tissue, Lymph nodes** and **Fascia**. This is in contrast with other authorities that insist the Spleen is related to muscles. The Stomach also deals with digestion in that it receives and stores food before releasing it to the small bowel. It is also related to **Connective Tissue**. When the stomach or spleen are in a state of imbalance there is sluggishness in the lymphatic circulation and fascia. The emotional counterparts of the Earth Element are **Empathy, Sympathy, Worry** and **Depression**. The Spleen also controls clear energy to the head, thus giving a clear head. Impairment of spleen energy will result in **Muzzy Headedness**.

Metal Element – This Element consists of the **Lung** (yin) and **Large Intestine** (yang) organs. Lung energy controls breath intake and all aspects of this (sinuses etc.) as well as the **Skin** and **Hair**. The Large Intestine, naturally, is the main organ of excretion and rids the body of toxins. Regarding the spine, the Lung and Large Intestine energies control the flow of cerebrospinal fluid. The emotional counterpart of Lung energy is **Grief** and **Lack of Expression** whilst the Large Intestine energy deals with **Guilt, Sadness** and **Regret** and not coping with change or alteration.

The Table below summarises the effect of emotions on the spinal tissues based upon the Law of Five Elements

Element	Metal	Earth	Fire	Wood	Water
Organs	Lung Large Intestine	Stomach Spleen	Heart Pericardium Triple Energiser Small Intestine	Liver Gall Bladder	Kidney Bladder
Spinal Tissues	CSF Skin Hair	Lymphatics Connective and Fat Tissue Ligaments	Blood Vessels Circulation	Muscles Tendons	Vertebrae Nervous Systems
Emotions	Guilt, Sadness Regret	Empathy, Worry Sympathy Depression	Excess Joy Love Assimilation	Anger, Rage Irritability Resentment Frustration Irrational Behaviour	Fear Anxiety Phobias

The Sheng and Ko cycles

Figure 1.3.1 shows the diagrammatic representation of the Five Elements Law and how vital force may be transferred from one Element to another and from one organ to another via the Sheng (clockwise to the adjacent Element, or the Mother Nourishing Son) cycle or the Ko (clockwise skipping one Element, or the Grandmother Restraining Grandson). It is said that the Sheng cycle is the engendering cycle and the Ko cycle is one of balance or control (for every yang there is a yin). These are well known by acupuncturists who have studied Five Elements acupuncture (and *should* be well known by all acupuncturists). A little understood aspect of this amazing natural Law is the Reverse Ko cycle.

Reverse Ko Cycle – Whereas the Sheng and Ko cycles involve the transference of vital force (chi) around the body, the reverse Ko cycle deals with disease and how dis-ease, as a force, may be transferred from organ to organ and from system to system. The subject of how disease enters the body in the first place is a very complicated one and would need a book to explain in detail (now there's a thought!). Dis-ease as a force may enter the yang system of internal organs via accident, inoculation, virus, poison, emotion (and a hundred other ways). Disease Force is then transferred from organ and system by the reverse Ko cycle. An example would be disease force entering the small intestine through a virus or bacteria. Then if this infection is heavily suppressed with antibiotics and the vital force isn't strong enough to fight the invasion, the dis-ease is then transmitted along the reverse Ko cycle to the bladder. This would be in the form of cystitis or some other ailment. Once again if suppressive remedies are used, the disease – as a force – would then enter the stomach, then the gall bladder, large intestine and finally back to the small intestine. The dis-ease could then enter the Yin system, which is, of course, more serious and life dependent. Having interviewed hundreds of patients over the past forty years, I can vouch that this happens. One can trace the patient's illnesses throughout their lives. At any one time in our lives we are a summation of all the trials and tribulations that have befallen us. If each imbalance has been successfully tackled with natural remedies, then disease force will not progress, but if at each stage suppression has taken place and the vital force isn't strong enough to fight, then tissue changes will occur.

That is all well and good, you may say, but how does this affect the spine. The spine, obviously, does not exist in isolation to the rest of the body, so dis-ease may transfer from system to system within the Laws of the Five Elements. So, the disease force would 'travel' from, say, the fascia or connective (Earth) to the muscles (Wood) to the cerebrospinal fluid (Metal) to the blood circulation (Fire) and then to the vertebrae or skull (Water). Check this one out with your patients who have chronic spinal instability and you may see a pattern forming.

Other types of traditional approaches to medicine, such as Ayurveda, also state the importance of the mind and our emotions to the welfare of the spine. In Part Two of this book the chakra energy system is discussed in detail.

Mind Body Relationships
The mind and body interact constantly and are jointly responsible for all conditions of health and disease. Discounting the mind's ability to cause and cure pain is the crucial mistake made by both patients and doctors alike. This is one of the great failings of the Cartesian medical philosophy, which has ruled with an iron hand over healthcare for generations. It is just in recent years that most traditionally trained doctors are finally realizing the undeniable... that the mind can cause, contribute to and perpetuate pain and the mind can also help cure it.

Psychological back pain is real. The pain is not imaginary or exaggerated. Unlike injury or disease which has a purely anatomical causative process, the symptoms of psychosomatic conditions are sourced in the mind. However, the pain is not in the mind. The physical symptoms are actual and exist totally in the body. Numbness, tingling and weakness are real. The cause of these symptoms is also real. The cause of these conditions is not physical - it is psychological and emotional.

As practitioners, we have all met the chronically sick patient who has been to see everyone in attempt to ease their symptoms. We are usually their 'last resort'. They will come with the tale that because everyone else has been unable to 'cure' them, the final person for them to see would be the psychiatrist, because it is perceived that their condition is 'all in the mind'. We now know that there is more than a grain of truth in this, but not necessarily in the way that it is meant.

Science is beginning to discover the physical and chemical connections between emotional state and physical condition. There have now been dozens of chemicals isolated - known as neuropeptides. These are small protein chemicals that act in the nervous system as transmitters of information. But we are not just talking about knowledge, we are talking about feelings. Depending on what "soup" of these tiny hormones is running around inside of you right now pretty much reflects what you are feeling emotionally.

Most of us would assume that these neuropeptides – such as endorphins, adrenaline, serotonin, dopamine, opiates to name a few, 'live' in our brain. Our culture has restricted the concept of emotions to never venture south of the skull and to be 'of the brain'. We now realize that many of these chemicals live in the spinal cord, and some even can be found around the tiny cells all over and inside the body, including the gut and heart. What this means is that when you "feel" an emotion, your entire body is feeling it! We have all felt the sudden, almost painful sensations in the solar plexus region occurring in acute anxiety. Because this sensation may be so overwhelming, we don't usually feel discomfort anywhere else in the body. However, when acute anxiety becomes chronic anxiety syndrome, due to on-going stress, for example, we commence to feel pain, discomfort, paresthesia etc. in other parts of the body.

I am not convinced that many 'acute' conditions such as sprains, strains, muscle pulls, cramp etc. are attributed to the mind-body connection. These, in my mind (no pun intended) are mostly due to an over exertion of a certain part of the body that is already in a state of stress, either due to its own previous work load (repetitive strain syndrome) or its reflective part of the body being is under stress. Posture, alignment, lifestyle and occupation all have their role to play in the formation of an acute spinal anomaly. The standard ways of spinal condition diagnosis are X-ray, MRI or CT scan. These are mostly helpful but can fall short of being a benefit when one realizes that each is just a snap shot in time. Each does not describe the months or years of mechanical, chemical or emotional changes that have occurred in the patient to eventually reach the stage of symptoms being present. I have seen many X-rays of, say, lumbar spine that show little or no bony changes, yet the patient is in a great deal of pain. Conversely, I have also seen many X-rays of gross abnormal spines where no pain is felt. The only way to truly ascertain a lasting solution to the patient's symptoms is to find the *true* cause. Sadly, as physical therapists, it is not always within our professional practice limitations so to do, especially when there is obvious emotional aetiology. One must always be prepared to refer one's patient to another better qualified practitioner when there is obviously no improvement, when you feel there should be after your treatment regimen.

Mind Body Relationships with Chronic Spinal Conditions
Many chronic spinal conditions occur due to our previous traumas, childhood experiences, our personality and character and general lifestyle. We are what we are at any one time of our lives as a composite of that earlier life – mind, body and spirit. Our childhood illnesses and experiences have huge impacts on illnesses we have as adults, and because the spine is our central column, and linked with every other aspect of our body, it is the spine that falls foul of our previous experiences. Chronic spinal conditions such as spondylosis, lumbago, ankylosing spondylitis, scoliosis etc. don't just occur for no reason. These chronic conditions are merely the final point that your body has reached attempting to cope with the original imbalance within your system. The symptoms of these conditions is your attempt at showing the outside world what is occurring within. Symptoms are a form of expression – they are not the dis-ease itself.

Emotions or Belief Systems?
I have intimated that most chronic spinal conditions have their genesis years ago, long before things become symptomatic, due to occurrences in childhood or adolescence. Although there is an obvious difference between negative emotions and our belief systems, both tend to give us the same conditions. For this section of the book I shall discuss muscular, bony and joint imbalance and in Part Two, individual sections of the spine are covered.

Fibromyalgia affects muscles all around the body as well as spinal one. The old-fashioned term for fibromyalgia (fibrositis) of the lower spine is **lumbago**. Stiffness, pain and muscle spasm are the chief symptoms. In all chronic muscular imbalance, there is always a history of anger, irritability, resentment or frustration over a long period of time. Much of the anger comes from the inability to cope with expectations from others (at school, college etc.). So instead of having freedom within our muscles, they become tight as we attempt to express our mindset. Also with lumbago there may be sexual suppression, resulting in low libido or abstinence.   When the lumbar spine is stiff, there is always a tendency towards the person not being able to cope with the various travails of life.

Cervical Spondylosis is osteoarthritis in the cervical spine. When it becomes chronic it gives pain and paresthesia locally and down the arms, neck stiffness, shoulder pain and heavy and painful lower limbs. The 'wear and tear' of the cervical facet joints and the subsequent soft tissue changes may be caused by misalignment of any other aspect of the spine due to trauma as a reflective action. One of the main causes, however is long term stress causing the classic stooped posture of the lower cervical spine and shoulders. The stress involved is usually centred upon the suppression of emotions in childhood or adolescence. The inability to adequately express our emotions leads to many conditions centred around the lower neck and shoulder, such as 'frozen shoulder' and chronic capsulitis.

Ankylosing Spondylitis (AS) usually affects the lower lumbar and sacro-iliac joints. It is now recognized as being an autoimmune condition (like rheumatoid arthritis) where osseous tissue replaces ligaments in the spine, thus rendering the spine stiff and solid. Any chronic condition affecting the bony system is always due to suppressed or repressed fear. In my experience, people with AS usually have chronic bowel imbalance.

Scoliosis is where the spine is unnaturally curved in a lateral direction either as an 'S' or a long 'C' shape. It usually affects the mid thoracic spine and is a complicated condition. It may be a congenital abnormality or appear slowly at adolescence (adolescent or idiopathic scoliosis). If the latter, it is often accompanied by childhood unhappiness and suppression of emotions. It affects young girls more than boys and there appears to be a self-consciousness issue at the heart of its formation. The teenager may be unduly petite or heavy or have some other distinguishing abnormality that creates long term self-consciousness. This, itself is ironic, as when the abnormal spinal curve starts to form it produces more self-consciousness.

I appreciate, only too well, that many readers will violently disagree with my conclusions as to the aetiology of chronic spinal disease. My findings are based upon analysis (and subsequent treatment) of thousands of patients over a considerable length of time. I also appreciate that these two books are about the treatment of spinal conditions using acupressure, reflexology and other subtle bodywork techniques. You may be thinking, at this stage, that only the talking therapies of psychology, psychiatry plus meditation, yoga and other 'relaxing' forms of therapy are the only disciplines that will help if the cause of the condition is emotional. Let me assure you that subtle bodywork has the power to treat all spinal conditions irrespective of the aetiology. All this will be found in Part Two of Book Two.

PART TWO
Energetic Concepts of the Spine

Chapter Four – Spinal Energy Therapy Overview

Knowledge and interpretation of the subtle or energy body is just as important, if not more important, than knowledge and interpretation of the anatomy and physiology of the physical body. I make no apology whatsoever in saying this and do so with the experience of working with both the physical body and subtle body for over forty years. Our anatomical knowledge underpins our capacity to practice whatever form of medicine we use, be it osteopathy, physiotherapy, reflexology etc. and we would not be able to practice medicine without knowing the 'nuts and bolts' of the human frame. Once we gain knowledge of the subtle body however, a whole new world is opened to us and we wonder how on earth we managed to improve the lot of our patients and clients without it.

I qualified as a chartered physiotherapist in 1970 and for the first few years practiced sports and soft tissue medicine (as most male physios do). There was, though, the still small voice that was trying to tell me that 'surely there must be more to therapy than this' – I wanted to treat *more* than musculo-skeletal conditions but didn't know how. It was then that a fellow physiotherapist joined our department who had spent some time in the Far East. He tried to explain to me about acupuncture and told me he had adopted this seemingly crazy and bizarre form of medicine in treating a few of his patients - with good results. I knew instinctively that this approach was for me. I enrolled on the 1976 2-year Lic. Ac. course at the British College in London. It was one of the first courses of its kind to be run in the U.K. and, although there were many times during the 2 years that I almost gave up due to having to learn a completely foreign type of body physiology, I persevered and gained my certificate to practice in 1978. I was the first chartered physiotherapist to also be qualified as an acupuncturist. That was the beginning of my fascinating journey in complementary medicine knowledge where I completed a baccalaureate and doctorate in acupuncture as well as doing courses in homoeopathy, reflexology, craniosacral therapy and a whole host of other bodywork courses. Without doing the initial acupuncture course, my life would have taken quite a different road and I would never had realised the joy and satisfaction of writing and teaching others about subtle bodywork techniques. I did not question or doubt the efficacy of energy medicine because I knew it worked and, what is more important, so did my patients. There were, of course, many in my profession who not only refused to accept any form of therapy that hadn't been scientifically proven but were also downright antagonistic towards me and my chosen pathway. This is not the place to enumerate these but, one day, I may explain all the trials and tribulations that I had to withstand in those early days – and since!

In the 21st century, we take it for granted that each city, town and village has complementary medicine therapists plying their trade – be it osteopaths, chiropractors, reflexologists, healers, reiki practitioners, acupuncturists, homoeopaths and the like. Prior to the 1970's however, it was a very different story. I remember that when I qualified as an acupuncturist, there were only two other acupuncturists in the whole of Devon. For non-UK readers, Devon is the third largest county in England. How times have changed. I am unsure of the numbers of osteopaths and chiropractors countrywide fifty years ago, but it is a sure thing that numbers have proliferated. One just has to look at the number of professional associations of the individual professions to understand that energy medicine practice is now 'big business'.

The main energy therapy bodywork practices in the modern world are acupuncture, reflexology, osteopathy, chiropractic, healing, reiki and the several 'touch' therapies of acupressure, shiatsu, Bowen and craniosacral therapy. There are, of course, scores more therapies not mentioned but most them are interpretations by individual pioneers of the original ones. A vast number in the more 'orthodox' professions of medicine and physiotherapy also practise one or more complementary therapies. Below we shall discover the origins of the different professions who use their skills to treat spinal conditions – namely

Acupuncture/Acupressure, Reflexology, Osteopathy, Cranial Osteopathy, Craniosacral therapy, Chiropractic, Applied Kinesiology, Touch for Health, Polarity Therapy and Chakra Healing. There are scores more but space does not permit me to mention any others in detail.

Energy medicine (often called vibrational medicine or holistic medicine) has two main principles to which it adheres. Firstly, it states that all living matter has an invisible 'vital force' by which 'healing' occurs. Secondly, no distinction is made between mind and body in that structural imbalances are often caused by negative emotions. Vital Force has been given very many different names over the centuries. In traditional Chinese medicine, it is called *Chi*, traditional Indian (Ayurvedic) medicine calls it *Prana*, whilst traditional Japanese medicine pens it *Ki* and the ancient priests of Hawaii called it *Mana*. Hippocrates called it *Medicatrix Naturae*, Paracelsus named it *Archaeus*, Mesmer penned it *Animal Magnetism* and Von Reichenberg called it *Odic Force* (to name but a few). Modern Western or allopathic medicine is mechanistic in practice and generally treats (or suppresses) symptoms at the expense of not considering the whole person or the symptom's aetiology. Energy medicine insists that symptoms are the patient attempting to express energetic imbalance of their mind/body and that medicine should be geared to help create energy balance, thus easing the symptoms. Each person is capable of 'self-healing' using their own vital force and the practitioner merely provides the wherewithal to allow the patient to heal themselves. You would also be forgiven for thinking that the mechanistic practices of osteopathy and chiropractic didn't have energetic genesis – you would be wrong.

Acupuncture/Acupressure

Acupuncture provides a persuasive argument for the healing energy theory. Traditional acupuncture originated in India around 5,500 years ago, and was later spread to China, Egypt and Asia by Buddhist monks and was later transferred to Japan and other far Eastern countries. It was quaintly thought that warriors returning from war exhibiting spear and arrow wounds would slowly be healed of other conditions as their wounds healed, the site of the wound often having no bearing on the diseased part that improved. Over several decades, points were mapped out on the body that seemed to exert an influence on certain internal organs and other parts of the body if they were stimulated with finger pressure, bamboo needle or burning. These points were called *acupuncture points*, *acupoints*, *xue* or *tsubo*. Acupoints on the body that possessed a similar internal organic or bodily system affinity were 'joined together' in a series of invisible energy lines called meridians or channels. Each of the meridians was named after its corresponding organ or system. The meridians appeared to house the *Chi* and it was sedated or stimulated by treating the acupoint. There are 12 main bilateral meridians plus 2 unilateral ones. The bilateral meridians that influence internal organs are Large Intestine (LI), Small Intestine (SI), Stomach (ST), Gall Bladder (GB), Bladder (BL), Lung (LU), Heart (HT), Spleen (SP), Liver (LR), Kidney (KI) and Pericardium (PC). To this is added the Triple Energizer (TE) channel. The unilateral meridians are the Governor (Gov) and Conception (Con). The two components of *chi* are 'Yin' and 'Yang' – they are opposites and yet complementary to each other. Yin and Yang philosophy forms the backbone of traditional Chinese, Japanese, Indian and tribal medicines. The ideas behind them developed by observing the physical world. It was seen that nature appears to group into pairs of dependant opposites. Thus, the concept of 'night' has no meaning or relevance without the concept of 'day'. There is no such thing as absolute Yin or absolute Yang and an increment of one always appears in the other. The Yin meridians are positioned on the front and inner aspects of the body whilst that Yan meridians are on the back and outer aspects. There are literally hundreds of Yin and Yang associations but the ones that are most linked to the spine are as follows: -

Yin – Chronic pain and chronic conditions, Stiffness, Oedema, Vital Organs
Yang – Acute pain and acute conditions, Mobility, Inflammation, Hollow Organs.

The main two meridians associated with spinal imbalance are the Bladder (BL) and Governor (Gov) with Small Intestine (SI), Gall Bladder (GB) and Large Intestine (LI) also in the frame. These will be discussed in detail in the next chapter. This book deals with touch therapy in aiding spinal complaints. Acupressure has been around as long as acupuncture, in fact it precedes it. I have repeatedly said in print and in talks that acupressure is *not* a watered-down version of acupuncture. In many ways, it seems to be much more useful, especially in the treatment of musculo-skeletal conditions and, of course, the treatment of patients who have needle phobia. When performed correctly, it is just as effective as needle. Probably the biggest advantage of acupressure over acupuncture is that you get an immediate feedback from the patient as to exactly what is occurring within the tissues.

Reflexology

Reflexology has been practised for well over five thousand years and its roots seem to be the same as traditional Oriental medicine. The modern practice of 'zone therapy' began when an American E.N.T. specialist, Dr. William Fitzgerald noticed that when his patients performed his version of 'painful point therapy', their post-operative pain seemed to be much less than those of his patients who didn't do any post-operative work. He postulated that the body can be divided into ten equal sections (five on each side of the body) along its vertical plane from head to feet. These sections were not just skin deep but seemed to affect internal organs as well. An American masseuse, Eunice Ingham, interested in Dr, Fitzgerald's work, concentrated her efforts in mapping out both vertical and horizontal zones on the feet, as well as body points. She invented what is one of the most popular forms of reflexology, namely foot zonal therapy. Figure 1.4.1 shows the vertical and horizontal lines of 'force' on the feet and body.

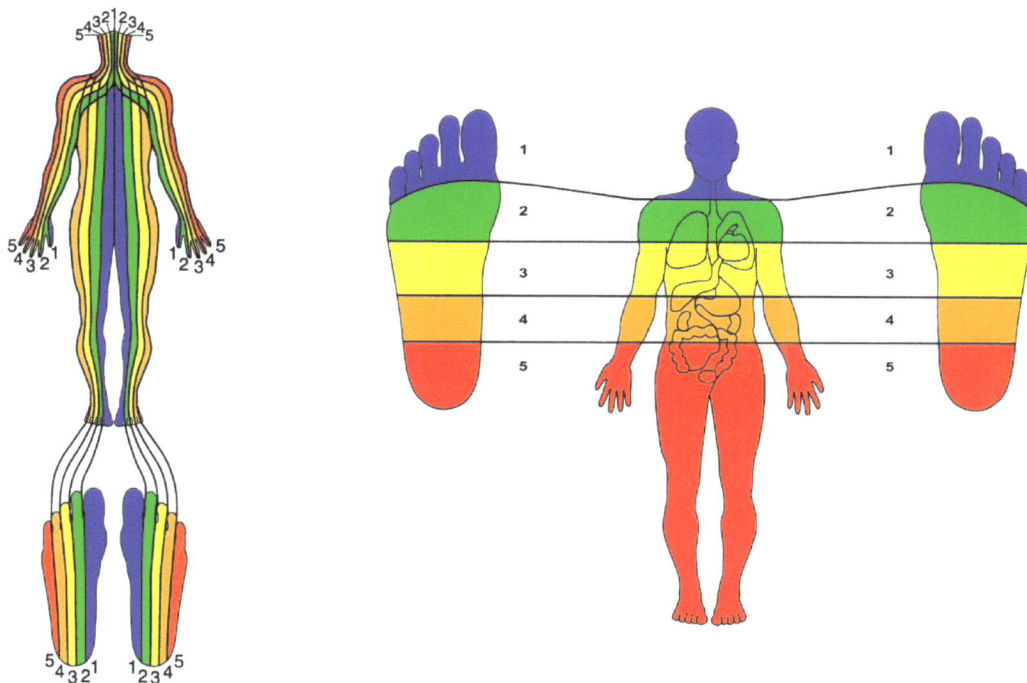

Figure 1.4.1 Vertical and Horizontal Body and Feet Zones

You can deduct from the vertical and horizontal zones illustration that the spine is situated in Zone 1 in the vertical and that, in the horizontal, the cranium and cervical spine is within Zone 1, the thoracic spine is within Zones 2 and 3, the lumbar spine is in Zone 4 and the sacrum/coccyx is situated in Zone 5. These various zones are extremely important in practical treatment terms and will be discussed fully in Book Two. There are very many approaches to reflexology, and, although it has its roots firmly in energy medicine, the practice these days tends to be mechanistic and rote in nature, with little reference to the energy body. I am a firm believer of using light touch and involving the client/patient as much as possible and consider it to be an integrated therapy as opposed to just digging the thumbs into the tender foot areas. This, and more will be covered in Book Two.

Osteopathy In 1874, Andrew Taylor Still MD DO (1828-1917), a medical doctor living on the Missouri frontier, discovered the significance of living anatomy in health and disease. Dr. Still realized that optimal health is possible only when all the tissues and cells of the body function together in harmonious motion. He reasoned that disease could have its origins in slight anatomical deviation from normal. He then proved he could restore health by treating the body with his hands, naming his innovative approach *osteopathy*. He understood that the human body is composed of many parts, all intimately related as a functional whole. More than a hundred years ago, Dr. Still realized that the human being is more than just a physical body. He envisioned a totally new medical system that acknowledges the relationships of the body, mind, emotions and spirit.

At the age of ten, young Andrew Still suffered from frequent headaches with nausea. He constructed a rope swing between two trees, eight to ten inches off the ground. He lay down using the rope for a swinging pillow. He wrote, "I lay stretched on my back, with my neck across the rope. Soon I became easy and went to sleep, got up in a little while with headache all gone." He continued to use this 'treatment' successfully every time he had a headache. Many years later Dr. Still considered his 'rope swing treatment' of headaches, and realized … "I had suspended the action of the great occipital nerves, and given harmony to the flow of the arterial blood to and through the veins…I have worked from the days of a child…to obtain a more thorough knowledge of the workings of the machinery of life, in producing ease and health."

As a practicing physician Dr. Still diligently researched and developed osteopathy. He discovered that he had the ability to treat patients with his hands, to change their physiology and restore health. In abbreviated form, the four tenets of Still's philosophy are: -

- The body functions as a total biological unit.
- The body possesses self-healing and self-regulatory mechanisms.
- Structure and function are interrelated.
- Abnormal pressure in one part of the body will produce abnormal pressures and strains in other body parts.

This was ground breaking stuff in the early 19th century, and Still never wavered from his principles of holistic medicine even though he suffered many personal tragedies that could have badly affected him. He is probably best known in non-osteopathic circles for his all-embracing phrase 'Structure Governs Function'

Cranial Osteopathy Still's most famous student, William Sutherland, was the grandson of a Scottish immigrant. He was born in Maine in 1873. In 1899, Sutherland was in his final year at Stills American School of Osteopathy in Kirksville. There was a collection of bone specimens mounted in a display case at the college, including a disarticulated skull. He stopped to look at it and was struck 'as if from a bolt from the blue' as he looked at the squamosal suture of the temporal bones, the rolling-overlap joint between the temporal and the parietal bone. He heard the words, 'Bevelled, like the gills of a fish, indicating articular mobility for a respiratory mechanism.' After graduating, Sutherland found himself strangely haunted by the experience. He tried to dismiss it, but it stayed with him. 'Forget it, you chump,' he kept telling himself. In the fifth year of practice, he could suppress his curiosity no longer, and pried apart a human skull with his penknife. It was a mark of his tactile skill that he did not break a single bone. He began to contemplate this jigsaw puzzle of parts. He kept this endeavour to himself, fearful of ridicule. He did not even tell his wife about his 'wild ideas.' On another occasion, by using leather straps around his head, he managed to stop all movement in both of his temporal bones. He noted with professional candour that he underwent 'personality changes.' His wife Adah noted that 'Such a strange sense of reality occurred that even when discussing it many years later, a shadow of the same altered reality again entered his consciousness.'

In 1925, with much trepidation and self-doubt, Sutherland gave his first cranial osteopathy lecture. In 1929 Sutherland sent his first article to the American Osteopathic Association. It was published that year and he would never think of turning back again. His short, poignant and masterful book, 'The Cranial Bowl' was published in 1939. In it, Sutherland wrote about an experiment upon himself that amounted to nothing less than advanced Raja Yoga. He was fond of saying, "Some of us do not have to go to sleep to see visions." Sutherland died in 1954, in his eighty-second year. He brought cranial osteopathy to the world. His "crazy thought" unfolded into a gift of healing. His was an enormous contribution. Modest to the end, Sutherland summed up his work thus: 'All I have done is pull aside a curtain for further vision. He recognized that the motion of cranial bones is connected to other tissues with which they are closely associated. The membrane system, which is continuous with cranial bones along their inner surfaces, is an integral part of this phenomenon. Significantly, Dr Sutherland also found that the central nervous system, and the cerebrospinal fluid which bathes it, have a rhythmic motion. The sacrum, too, is part of this interdependent system. Thus, there is an important infrastructure of fluids and tissues at the core of the body which express an interrelated subtle rhythmic motion.

As he dug deeper into the origins of these rhythms, he realized that there are no external muscular agencies which could be responsible. He concluded that this motion is produced by the body's inherent life-force itself, which he called the *Breath of Life*. This was seen by Dr Sutherland to be the animator or spark behind these involuntary rhythms. Alluding to the source of this phenomenon, other practitioners have referred to it as "the soul's breath in the body". The Breath of Life is considered to carry a subtle yet powerful "potency" or force, which produces subtle rhythms as it is transmitted around the body. Dr Sutherland realized that the cerebrospinal fluid has a significant role in the expressing and distributing the potency of the Breath of Life. As potency is taken up by the cerebrospinal fluid, it generates a tide-like motion which is described as its *longitudinal fluctuation*. This motion has great importance in carrying the Breath of Life throughout the body and, if it is expressed, health will follow.

Craniosacral Therapy In the mid-1970s Dr John Upledger was the first practitioner to teach some of these therapeutic skills to people who were not osteopathically trained. Dr Upledger had become drawn to exploring primary respiratory motion after an incident that occurred while he was assisting during a spinal surgical operation. He was asked to hold aside a part of the dural membrane system which enfolds the spine, while the surgeon attempted to remove a calcium growth. To his embarrassment, Dr Upledger was unable to keep a firm hold on the membrane, as it kept rhythmically moving under his fingers. He took a post-graduate course in cranial osteopathy and then set out on his own path of clinical research. Over the years, Dr Upledger has done a great deal to popularise craniosacral work around the world. When Dr Upledger began to teach non-osteopaths, he encountered great opposition from many in the profession who believed that the foundation of a full osteopathic training is necessary to practise the craniosacral approach. Many osteopaths are still of this opinion, and it continues to be a cause of much debate and argument. However, many also believe that this work can provide an integrated approach to health care and need not remain within the sole domain of osteopathic practice. Nevertheless, one thing is for sure - a good foundation in anatomy and physiology is necessary to apply craniosacral work with safety and competency. It was Dr Upledger who coined the term "craniosacral therapy" when he started to teach to a wider group of students. Dr Upledger wanted to differentiate the therapeutic approaches he had developed and, furthermore, the title "cranial osteopath" could not be used by those new practitioners who were not osteopathically trained.

One question frequently asked is, "What is the difference between cranial osteopathy and craniosacral therapy?" Although Dr Upledger states that these two modalities are different, the differences are not always so obvious. They both emerge from the same roots and have much common ground, yet different branches have developed. A variety of therapeutic skills are now commonly used by both osteopaths and non-osteopathic practitioners of this work, so neither cranial osteopathy nor craniosacral therapy can be accurately defined by just one approach. However, in practice, craniosacral therapists often work more directly with the emotional and psychological aspects of disease. It also tends to be much more gentle and subtle than cranial osteopathy.

Chiropractic The word 'Chiropractic' comes from the Greek words *cheir* (meaning 'hand') and *praktos* (meaning 'done'), i.e. Done by Hand. The name was chosen by the developer of chiropractic, Daniel David Palmer. A prolific reader of all things scientific, DD Palmer realized that although various forms of manipulation had been used for hundreds, if not thousands of years, no one had developed a philosophical or scientific rationale to explain their effects. Palmer's major contribution to the health field was therefore the codification of the philosophy, art and science of chiropractic which was based on his extensive study of anatomy and physiology.

Palmer performed the initial chiropractic adjustment in September 1895. He examined a janitor who had become deaf 17 years prior after he felt something "give" in his back. Palmer examined the area and gave a crude "adjustment" to what was felt to be a misplaced vertebra in the upper spine. The janitor then observed that his hearing improved. From that first adjustment, DD Palmer continued to develop chiropractic and in 1897 established the Palmer School of Cure, now known as the Palmer College of Chiropractic, in Davenport, Iowa, where it remains today. Following the first adjustment, many people became interested in Palmer's new science and healing art. It is now practiced worldwide.

Palmer discovered that disease is caused by abnormal functioning of the nervous system and that normal function is restored by manipulation of the spine (as well as other regions of the body). The nervous system becomes awry when vertebrae go out of alignment – known as a *subluxation,* resulting from bad posture, accidents, stress, poor diet or, indeed, any of the scores of causes outlined in this book. When the chiropractor adjusts the vertebra back to alignment, this creates harmony in the system and allows the body's own healing energy to flow impeded. Patients who have received adjustments often feel a 'rush of energy' up and down the spine that seemingly affects both physical and mental health. D.D. Palmer believed in a vital force that he called *Innate*. He was also interested in magnetic healing and wrote the following "All observers realize that we are surrounded with an aura: that we pass from our bodies a subtle, invisible substance known as magnetism; that this emanation may be either repellent or attractive. Heat, magnetism, odour, and no doubt other unseen force emanate from our bodies in all directions."

Palmer apparently believed that this energy-giving life to the body was 'nerve' force; that it was generated in the cells of the brain and the spinal cord and then sent out through the system of nerves to give power to the organs, as electricity is sent out through wires to furnish light, power and heat. His goal was to prove that disease of any organ may arise from defects of the nerve centres, rather than the organ itself.

Although this book is about the spine and therapies that treat it, it would be remiss not to briefly mention the two main 'offshoots' of chiropractic, namely Applied Kinesiology and Touch for Health – both of which purport to have many approaches and techniques in the treatment of spinal conditions.

Applied Kinesiology (AK) Traditionally, the word "kinesiology" refers simply to the study of muscles and body movement. In 1964, however, American chiropractor George J. Goodheart founded what has become known as 'applied' kinesiology when he linked oriental ideas about energy flow in the body with western techniques of muscle testing. First, Goodheart noted that all muscles are related to other muscles. He observed that for each movement a muscle makes, there is another muscle or group of muscles involved with that movement; one muscle contracts while another one relaxes. So, when he was presented with a painful, overly-tight muscle, he would observe and treat the opposite, and necessarily weak, muscle to restore balance. This was, 53 years ago, a very new technique. Applied kinesiology is based on the idea that the body is an interacting unit made of different parts that interconnect and affect each other. Everything we do affects the whole body, therefore, a problem in one area can cause trouble in another area. According to kinesiology, the muscles eventually register and reflect anything that is wrong with any part of the body, whether physical or mental. Thus, a digestive problem might show up in the related and corresponding muscles of the legs. By testing the strength of certain muscles, the kinesiologist claims to be able to gain access to the body's communication system, and, thus, to read the health status of each of the body's major components.

The manual testing of muscles or muscle strength is not new, and was used in the late 1940s to evaluate muscle function and strength and to assess the extent of an injury. Applied kinesiology measures whether a muscle is stuck in the "on" position, acting like a tense muscle spasm, or is stuck "off," appearing weak or flaccid. It is called manual testing because it is done without instruments, using only the kinesiologist's fingertip pressure. During the first and longest appointment, which lasts about an hour, the kinesiologist conducts a complete consultation, asking about the patient's history and background. During the physical examination, patients sit or lie down, then the kinesiologist holds the patient's leg or arm to isolate a particular muscle. The practitioner then touches a point on the body which he believes is related to that muscle, and, with quick, gentle, and painless pressure, pushes down on the limb. Patients are asked to resist this pressure, and, if they cannot, an imbalance is suspected in the related organ, gland, or body part. This diagnostic technique uses muscles to find the cause of a problem, and is based on traditional Chinese medicine and its idea that the body has common energy meridians, or channels, for both organs and muscles. Kinesiologists also claim that they can locate muscle weaknesses that stem from a variety of causes such as allergies, mineral and vitamin deficiencies, as well as from problems with the lymphatic system. Once the exact cause is determined, the kinesiologist uses his/her fingertips to work the appropriate corresponding acupressure points to rebalance the flow of energy and restore health.

Touch for Health (TFH) This practice became an offshoot of AK in the mid 1970's. I was one of the first to learn this form of therapy in the UK under Brian Butler. He had studied in the USA under John Thie DC. It uses the same principles as AK, but was meant for the non-chiropractic professions. It was somewhat castigated by professional therapists in that it was taught to lay people. On a personal level, I have never been persuaded to practice either AK or TFH as it just wasn't my 'thing'. Certain of its principles, though, I believe to be brilliant, especially the holistic approach of muscles, the reflected regions, dietary advice and the integration of other disciplines into their philosophy. I am not so sure about the so called 'neuro-vascular' points and the sheer validity of muscle testing. I believe that muscle testing should not be central to its practice as it cannot be replicated from practitioner to practitioner or even by the individual therapist in the same treatment session. Also, I believe that the therapy is only as good as the practitioner who performs it and I have witnessed several dire practitioners who have done some bandwagon jumping in attempting to learn a 'package' of therapeutic skills without having the underlying anatomical knowledge to practice safely. I have therefore, over the years, extracted from its wealth of teaching what I consider to be good practice and with which I am comfortable. That the therapy is only as good as the practitioner can, obviously, be said about any therapy and it is a good job that we are all different (and 'thick skinned' when one is condemned by others for not agreeing with them).

Polarity Therapy is a multidisciplinary approach to health and well-being. The father of Polarity Therapy, Dr. Randolph Stone, was born in Austria in 1890 and, after his mother's death, emigrated with his father to the USA in 1903. He studied religion and through a scholarship became a Lutheran minister. He soon realized that orthodox religion could not satisfy his spiritual needs and began studying many tomes by great spiritual leaders of the past. After taking a few months of solitary meditation he decided to study osteopathy, chiropractic and naturopathy and started a practice in Chicago. He also studied many ancient systems of healing such Ayurveda and Yoga and, eventually pioneered a therapy that he coined Polarity Therapy. He understood that 'all is energy' and that illness occurs when our energy (vital force) does not have free flow and when there are 'blockages' in both the physical and emotional. His far-reaching therapy is designed upon many different factors – TCM, the Chakras, Magnetism, Osteopathy, Cerebrospinal fluid flow, Reflexology and Nutrition. It is truly a holistic practice – but takes many months, if not years, to learn to a respectable level. There aren't many therapies that have combined so many different philosophies into one, understandable and repeatable whole. Please read about his work with the Law of Five Elements – it answers much about why we become ill and have so many energy imbalances. He is a true pioneer in the understanding of complementary medicine and we all owe him a great debt. One of his quotes is "Health is not merely of the body. It is the natural expression of the body, mind and soul when they are in rhythm with the One Life. True health is the harmony of life within us, consisting of peace of mind, happiness and well-being. It is not a question of physical fitness, but is rather a result of the soul finding free expression through the mind of the individual" – Brilliant! Figure 1.4.2 shows how Dr. Stone thought that electromagnetic currents are said to flow continuously within and around the body. Note how it resembles Figure 2.1.1 and the chakra illustrations in a later chapter.

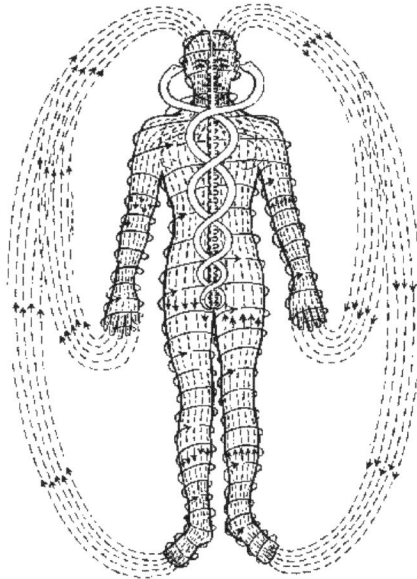

Figure 1.4.2 Polarity Therapy – based on Dr. Randolph Stone's work

Spinal Harmonics

Polarity Therapy is an all-encompassing approach to energy balancing the whole body, based on many different philosophies. A specific vertebral spin-off from Polarity Therapy is *Spinal Harmonics*. Randolph Stone found that vertebrae fell into groups of three, called 'spinal harmonics', as shown in Figure 1.4.3. An exception to the vertebral triad is the quartet of Sphenoid – T1 – T10 – Coccyx. When a vertebra is in a state of acute pain or congestion, contact is made with the spinal process of that vertebra, together with another vertebra in its triad. So, for instance, pain around C3 may be relieved by contacting T5 or L3. Light touch, focus and intention are required, often for a few minutes. If the patient is relatively relaxed (apart from the localised pain), it is possible for pain to be relived and realignment may occur if the cause of the pain/spasm was due to a facet lock. There is also an improvement in the energetic influence on the associated internal organ served by the vertebra. In my experience of performing this procedure, the treatment resolution falls into two different types: -

1. After some length of time keeping the fingers in situ (fully explained in Book Two), there is a spontaneous resolution when the pain and spasm ease whilst the patient remains still. The therapist feels this release at the same time as the patient.
2. The same hold with the finger pads as before, only this time the patient will begin to slowly 'unwind'. This may begin as a gradual spinal 'wriggling' and movement that sometimes becomes whole body 'writhing' as the self-healing of the patient is occurring (the practitioner is just to conduit). This may go on for some considerable time if the lesion is chronic and it may be difficult to keep contract with the spinous processes. (Again, this process is fully discussed in Book Two)

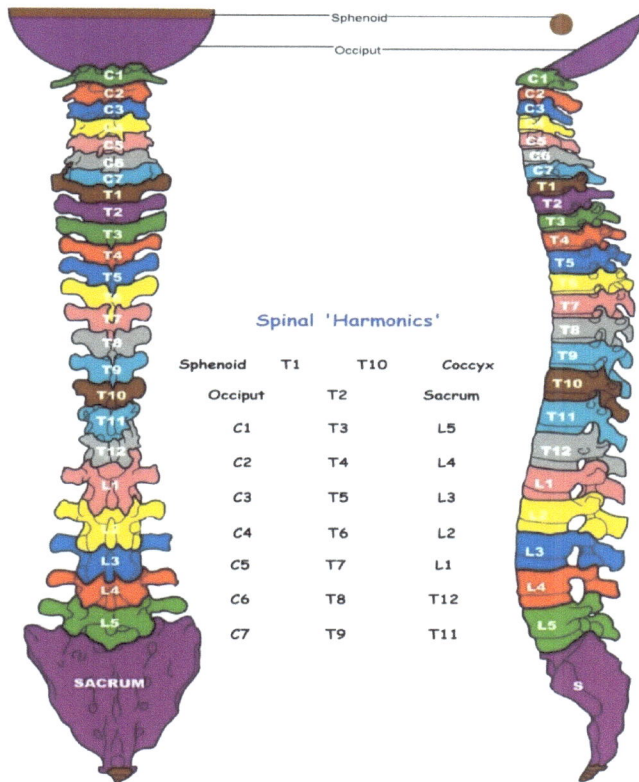

Spinal 'Harmonics'

Sphenoid	T1	T10	Coccyx
Occiput	T2		Sacrum
C1	T3		L5
C2	T4		L4
C3	T5		L3
C4	T6		L2
C5	T7		L1
C6	T8		T12
C7	T9		T11

Figure 1.4.3 Spinal Harmonics in Polarity Therapy

The Chakra Energy System

This ancient system of medicine is originally part of Ayurveda and is thousands of years old. It has stood the test of time as it is still practiced worldwide including its country of origin – India. I have spent the past four decades in the study and practice of this system of energy medicine and it has been a great privilege to have disseminated my knowledge to others. I am very pleased that this system is now practiced including 'physical' therapy, as it was only used to be discussed alongside meditation and yoga. This system and its affiliation to the spine will be discussed in full later.

Chapter Five – Meridians, Acupoints and Trigger Points

Before discussing the specific meridians and acupoints that are associated with the spine (and spinal conditions), it is necessary to attempt to quantify exactly what meridians and acupoints are. There have been many attempts at defining the true nature of the meridian by those who do not wish to look at them in the traditional Eastern way of them being invisible lines of force that enable chi energy to flow.

Traditional Views

Traditional Chinese medicine (TCM) describes meridians as a complex system of channels that carries energy (chi), blood and fluids around the body. They obviously operate at a subtle level and should be looked at as a process or system as opposed to having structural (tube like) form. The channels have high concentrations of chi that can be detected by one of a plethora of gadgets on the market that 'light up' their LED light when centrally over a meridian or acupoint and do not light up when away from the channels. Another traditional viewpoint sees the meridians as the 'etheric energy aspect' within the 'physical aspect' and considers the invisible (visible to clairvoyants) aura that surrounds us all. Acupoints are the focal points of energy that are mostly found along the meridian (although there are very many non-meridian acupoints). They are also known as *xue* or *tsubo* as well as *trigger points* or *reflex* points. The acupoint is where the chi energy can be sedated or stimulated and may be influenced by needle, pressure or moxa in allowing free flow of energy in the channel. They are often equated as being like lock gates on a canal system and when the lock gate is opened it allows the water to flow freely. In his book, *Complete Chinese Medicine* (Parragon 1996), Tom Williams likened acupoints as energy vortices that draw chi into or out of the body's energy flow providing access points whereby the chi flow of the body can be directly influenced by these vortices. Figure 1.5.1 shows how the acupoint can be compared to a miniature whirlpool or vortex, through which energy can be drawn. It is, indeed, a micro-chakra and this is something that I have believed for many years.

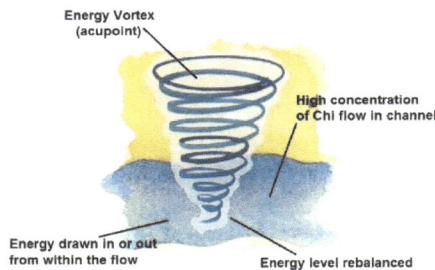

Energy Vortex
(acupoint)

High concentration
of Chi flow in channel

Energy drawn in or out
from within the flow

Energy level rebalanced

Figure 1.5.1 Comparing an acupoint to a miniature whirlpool/vortex

Parragon copyright – with thanks

Modern Views

Some meridians are positioned adjacent to major motor nerves and can mimic the effect of those nerves. Two that come to mind are the lower part of the Bladder meridian that mimics the sciatic nerve and the Heart meridian that is adjacent to the ulnar nerve. It is obvious to me that the meridian system (as well as most other systems in the body) are connected to or part of the central nervous system – they must be! Meridian channels aren't just on the surface of the body but are complex systems that include the surface channels (musculo-tendinous) and the deeper channels that 'connect' the internal organ or system to the superficial channels and major acupoints. Recently scientists at Seoul National University confirmed the existence of meridians, which they refer to as the "primo-vascular system." They say that this system is a crucial part of the cardiovascular system. Previously, North Korean scientist Kim Bong-Han proposed that he had found meridians in the early 1960's. Dr Kim Bong-Han showed over 50 years ago, that new tubular structures exist inside and outside of blood vessels and lymphatic vessels, as well as on the surface of internal organs and under the dermis. He believed they were the traditional meridian lines. The meridians were called Bonghan ducts or channels, after his research, but now the existence of this system in various organs has been corroborated by further research.

The Korean scientists studying oriental medicine with biophysical methods injected a special staining dye which coloured the meridians. By injecting the dye onto acupuncture points, they could see thin lines. These did not show up at non-acupuncture point sites where there are no meridians. The researchers discovered that the meridian lines are not confined to the skin, but are in fact a concrete duct system through which liquid flows, and that this liquid aggregates to form stem cells. Previously, scientists used a combination of imaging techniques and CT scans to observe concentrated points of microvascular structures that clearly correspond to the map of acupuncture points created by Chinese energy practitioners in ancient times. In a study published in the Journal of Electron Spectroscopy and Related Phenomena, researchers used contrast CT imaging with radiation on both non-acupuncture points and acupuncture points. The CT scans revealed clear distinctions between the non-acupuncture point and acupuncture point anatomical structures. Other studies have deducted that the complex meridian system is part of the various layers and levels of connective tissue within the body. Some major acupoints and trigger points appear to be nodes and nodules associated with the lymphatic system. Thomas Myers in his book 'Anatomy Trains' purported that the meridian system of the body lay within the fascial tissue and that as the body's fascia connects every part of the body in an integrated way, the meridians follow suit. It is understood that the acupoint (or trigger, reflex point) is a small region underneath the dermis that shows a lower electrical resistance compared with its surrounding tissues. They are undoubtedly linked to the central nervous system. It has been proved ad nauseam that pain relief acupuncture works by the release of endorphins from the brain but so far there is little scientific evidence of how acupuncture works where the relief of pain isn't an issue e.g. some internal organic and emotional conditions.

Meridians/Acupoints associated with the Spine

The main two meridians are the Governor and Bladder channels, with the Gall Bladder, Small Intestine and Large Intestine meridians having some influence on the spine. Figure 1.5.2 shows a diagrammatic representation of the spinal meridians – they are, of course, not straight lines – nothing in the body is – but the meridian lines 'join up' acupoints belonging to the same system or internal organ, and they are usually represented as being straight. Also, please note that my diagrams include the deeper pathways as well as the more superficial musculo-tendinous meridians. This will appear quite different to the traditional views of meridians – however, I feel that in showing the complete picture of each meridian, it gives a fuller picture and makes more sense as to why certain meridians are involved with certain conditions. On this illustration, the deep meridians are shown as solid lines – whereas in later illustrations they are shown as broken lines. A broken line in this illustration indicates that two meridians share the same pathway. You will also notice that there is a great confluence of meridian energy around the lower cervical region at Gov 14 and around the lower lumbo-sacral region.

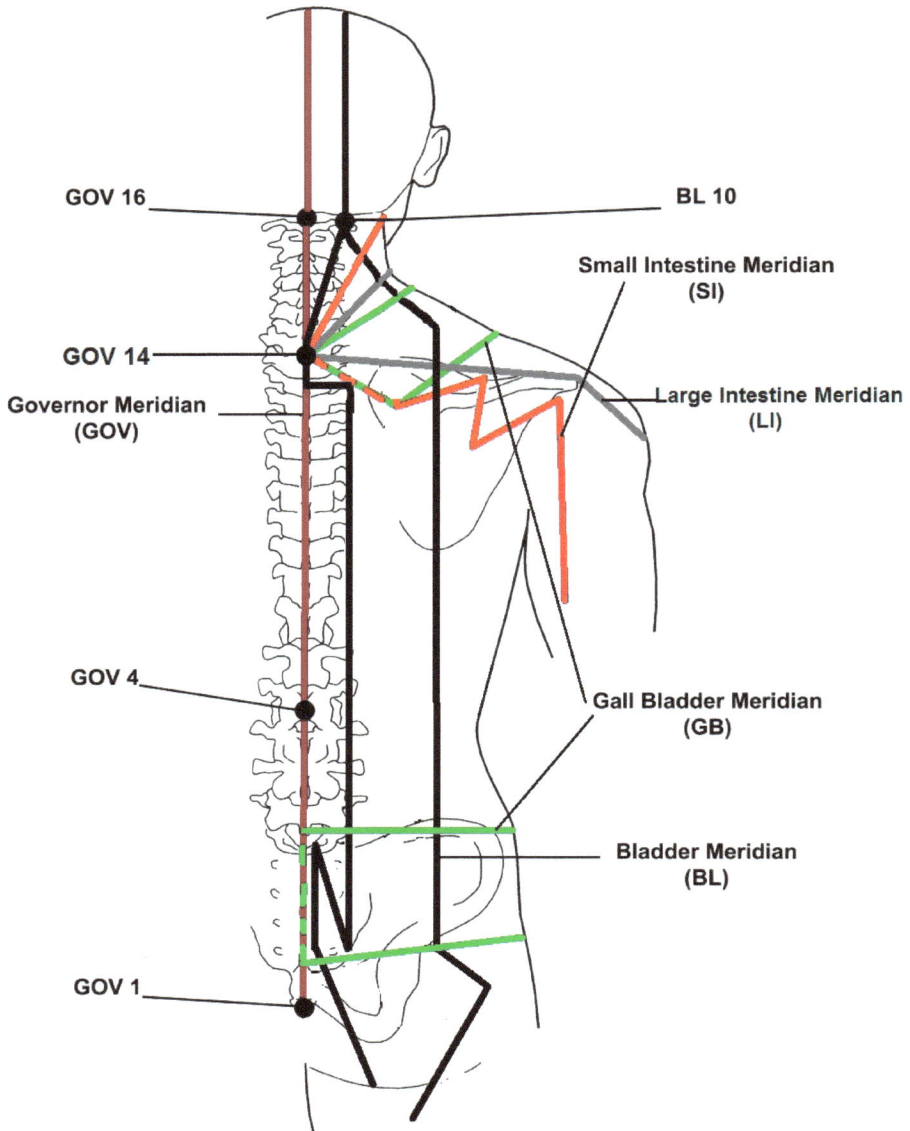

Figure 1.5.2 – Diagrammatic Representation of the Spinal Meridians

Governor Meridian

The Governor meridian is also known as the Du Mai, Governing or Steering channel. It is a Yang channel with its counterpart being the Conception channel which is Yin in nature. There are twenty-eight (28) acupoints along its surface pathway starting at the distal end of the coccyx and ending on the underside of the top lip. It is one of two unilateral meridians – the other being the Conception meridian that is aspected on the front line of the body. The meridian ascends directly up the midline of the spine and is the equivalent of the Sushumna Nadis in Ayurvedic philosophy (described in the next chapter). In every meridian, there are important and most used acupoints and the lesser and least used ones. The most used

50

ones by acupuncturists and other therapists are the points that have been shown to have more power and yield better results in treatment. In the bilateral meridians, the important, or Command points, lie between the limb extremity and the elbow/knee – this is where chi is moved. Naturally this does not occur on the Governor as the unilateral channel lies on the torso and head. The important acupoints on this channel are those that correspond to the posterior major chakras – these will be stated in this chapter and described in full in the next. The Governor channel is one of the eight extraordinary channels that has a designated 'key' point – used to 'open' the energy. This is acupoint SI 3, situated on the ulnar surface of the hand.

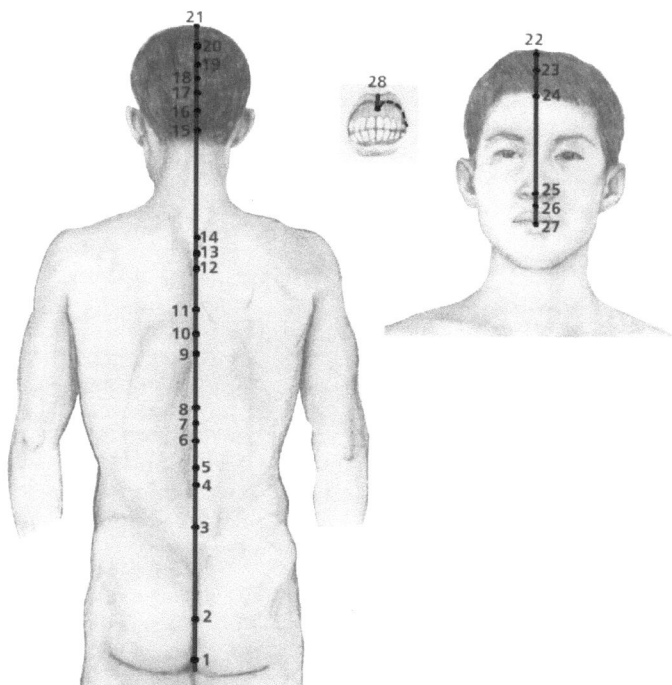

Figure 1.5.3 Governor Meridian

The following will be described in more detail as used in acupressure and acupuncture – Gov 1; Gov 2; Gov 3; Gov 4; Gov 14; Gov 16

Gov 1 – Situated between the tip of the coccyx and the anus. For obvious reasons this acupoint is not utilised much in acupressure, but with needle it is used to treat prolapsed rectum, haemorrhoids, constipation and painful urination. It is, though, considered to be the Muladhara (Base) chakra and, as such, is possibly the most important acupoint on the body.

Gov 2 – Situated in the midline between the sacrum and coccyx. Treats symptoms as per Gov 1 and is also used as the Base chakra in acupressure.

Gov 3 – Situated below the spinous process of L4. I considerl this acupoint the posterior aspect of the Sacral chakra and is therefore indicated in gynaecological conditions as well as oedema in the legs.

Gov 4 – Situated below the spinous process of L2. It is level with BL 23 and on the same girdle as the umbilicus. The TCM word for the point is *Ming Men* which means *Door of Life*. That is how important this acupoint is - it is an excellent acupoint with needle, pressure and moxa in the treatment of tiredness and lethargy as it is strongly related to kidney energy.

Gov 14 – Situated below the spinous processes of C7-T1. What an important acupoint! It is extensively used in acupuncture in the treatment of musculo-skeletal conditions, but it may be use for so much more. It lies at the centre of a parallelogram of forces with one axis being the spine and the other being the horizontal line between the shoulders. The area is therefore very prone to physical stress and tension. This acupoint is also the intersection of five meridians (some by deeper channels) so it is influential in conditions allied to the large intestine, small intestine, gall bladder and bladder as well as locally through the governor. These include

- Pain and stiffness of the neck, upper back, trapezius spasm, fibromyalgia and kyphosis
- Colds, fever, cough and sore throat, wheezing and chest conditions.
- Palpitations, tachycardia, mental restlessness, poor concentration and memory.
- Headache, migraine, hypertension and eye conditions.
- Bladder irritation, frequency
- Constipation, inability to express emotions, shyness

It is also said to be the posterior aspect of the Throat chakra – see next chapter

Gov 16 – Situated directly below the external occipital protuberance, in the depression between the attachments of the trapezius muscle. This very important acupoint is used mainly in conditions affecting the brain, head and mind. These include some symptoms of hemiplegia, aphasia, dizziness, headache, migraine, vertigo, blurred vision, epistaxis, tinnitus, dyspnoea, mental confusion, restlessness, agitation, insomnia and anxiety. Once more this point is said to be the posterior aspect of a major chakra – this time the Ajna (Brow) chakra. Together with its anterior counterpart (Yintang – between the eyebrows), they are two very important acupoints in the treatment of stress and tension and for calming the mind. This especially works well in acupressure either on the patient or as self-treatment.

Bladder meridian

The Bladder meridian is the Yang channel in the Water Element. It is the longest meridian in the body with sixty-seven (67) points. It has a huge range of influences that vary according to the position of its acupoints. The surface meridian commences at the inner canthus of the eye before ascending and over the head, via Gov 24, then just lateral to the midline to BL 10 at the lateral aspect of the atlas. Here it divides into two meridians that are relatively parallel to the spine and to each other – these are commonly called the 'Inner' and 'Outer' bladder channels. The Inner channel firstly deviates to join with Gov 14 and Gov 13 before descending 1.5 cun laterally to the spine as far as the lower end of the sacrum. Here it almost reverses its direction to ascend medially to BL 31 at the first sacral foramen where it reverses again to descend through the sacrum to the lower end of the buttock, down the posterior aspect of the thigh to the popliteal fossa where it joins the outer channel at BL 40 in the centre of the popliteal fossa. Meanwhile the Outer channel leaves BL 10 at the occiput and descends roughly 3 cun parallel to the midline (Governor meridian) through the buttock and to the centre of the popliteal fossa at BL 40, deviating slightly to join GB 30 at the greater trochanter of the hip. At BL 23 and BL 52 a deep channel (not shown) travels to both the kidney and the bladder. Meanwhile the surface pathway at BL 40 descends the calf to the lateral aspect of the lower leg towards the lateral malleolus where it travels along the lateral aspect of the foot before ending at the nail of the little toe. The Bladder meridian along the spine is the equivalent of the Ida and Pingala Nadis in Ayurveda. As you can imagine this meridian is generally broken into sections to describe it fully. These are the Head; The Inner Bladder line; The Outer Bladder line; The Sacral points and the

Leg/Foot points. We shall describe the middle 3 as they have most relevance to the spine, but the practical chapter will describe some of the Leg/Foot points as they are used in the treatment of spinal conditions.

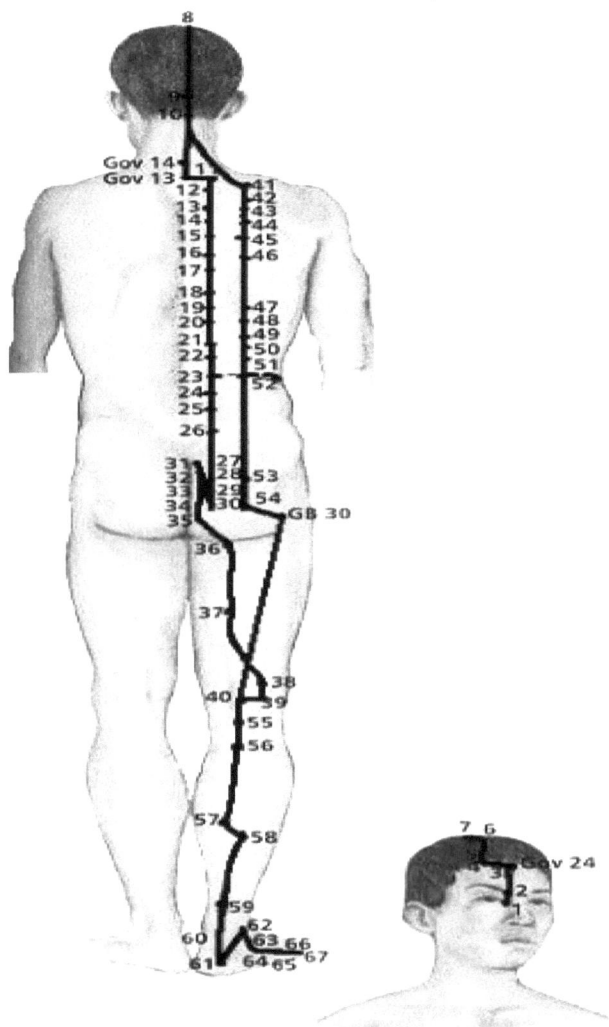

Figure 1.5.4 The Bladder meridian

The Inner Bladder Line

The Inner Bladder Line houses the wonderful 'Back Transporting Points'. These are also known as the 'Associated Effect Points' or the 'Back-Shu' Points. This section of the bladder meridian travels from the lateral aspect of T1 (BL 11) down to S2 (BL28). All the acupoints on this section are situated 1.5 cun (two fingers width) lateral to the midline, at the highest part of the erector spinae (longissimus) muscle. Figure 1.5.5 refers. I well remember that whilst I was training in acupuncture (in the mid 1970's), the Inner Bladder Line made for riveting study and it was this, along with the Law of Five Transformations, that convinced me of the efficacy of acupuncture and the way that it could be integrated with modern therapies. It is said that these 15 acupoints transport chi to the internal organs and systems. Not only do they have an affinity for the organs but for the correspondences of the organs – these will be explained as they are enumerated below. These acupoints have also been called Spinal Reflex points as they may be used in acupressure and reflexology in analysis as well as treatment modalities. These points are mostly used in the treatment of chronic illness, but not exclusively to them. I have used them scores of times, with both acupuncture and acupressure in the treatment of acute maladies. They appear to be closely associated with the Sympathetic Nervous System (described in Part One and later in this chapter) in that each acupoint is anatomically adjacent to the point where the autonomic nerves emerge from the spine. In Figure 1.5.11 there is a correlation of the Inner Bladder Line, Outer Bladder Line and the Autonomic Nervous System

BL 11 – Great Shuttle – 1.5 cun lateral to the lower border of the spinous process of **T1**

This acupoint doesn't seem to be mentioned much in acupuncture tomes and certainly not as a Back-Transporting Point, and is insignificant– I must disagree! It is used to treat cervical and occipital stiffness and pain, sore throats and occipital headaches. The most important fact about this point is that it is the master point of any disorder associated with bone and bony conditions. It should therefore be used (in conjunction with other points) in osteoporosis, kyphosis, scoliosis, osteoarthritis, ankylosing spondylosis and where there is difficulty in fractures uniting. I have always assumed that the point stimulates the parathyroid glands (level with this point at the front of the neck) though have never read this anywhere; the anatomical juxtaposition is too much of a coincidence.

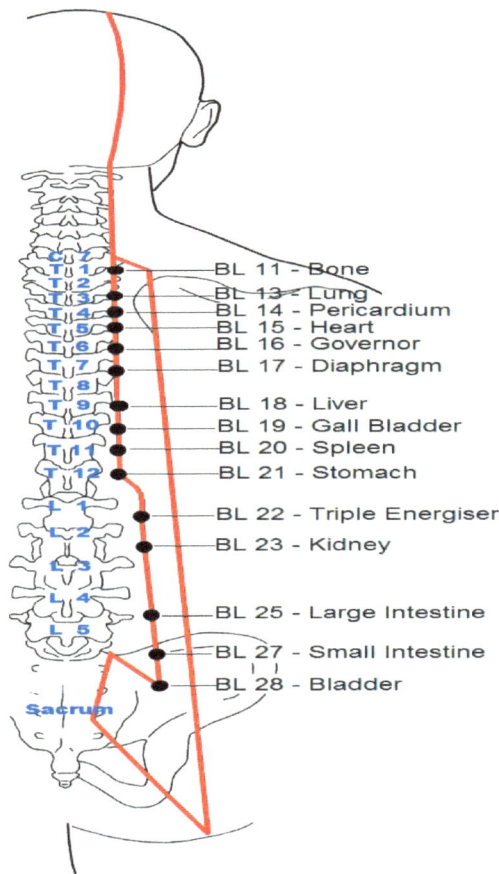

Figure 1.5.5 The Back-Transporting Points of the Inner Bladder Line

BL 13 – Lung Shu Point - 1.5 cun lateral to the lower border of the spinous process of **T3**

This acupoint is used in all manner of lung conditions. Symptoms include acute or chronic cough, sore throat, acute and chronic respiratory conditions, nasal congestion, chronic tiredness and night sweats.

BL 14 – Pericardium Shu Point – 1.5 cun lateral to the lower border of the spinous process of **T4**

This acupoint regulates pericardium, heart and liver chi and is used to treat chest congestion, thoracic oppression, dyspnoea, retching and vomiting – also used as a local point in thoracic pain.

BL15 – Heart Shu Point – 1.5 cun lateral to the lower border of the spinous process of **T5**

This acupoint is used to nourish, cool and soothe the heart and is therefore an excellent point for arrhythmia, chest oppression, angina, vomiting and general circulatory conditions.

BL 17 – Diaphragm Shu Point – 1.5 lateral to the lower border of the spinous process of **T7**

This acupoint doesn't appear to have much influence on the diaphragm, even though in TCM it is the diaphragm Shu point. It is used, though, in abdominal tension, distension and pain. The main action of this acupoint is in the treatment of 'blood' related disorders. It is used to invigorate blood and dispel stasis as well as arresting bleeding. It is a well-known first aid point in the arrest of bleeding. In my experience, there is limited action on the treatment of hiccoughs.

BL 18 – Liver Shu Point – 1.5 cun lateral to the lower border of the spinous process of **T9**

Please note that no acupoints exist on the midline or the bladder channel at the level of T8, therefore the Transporting Points appear to skip a vertebra. This is an excellent acupoint in controlling chi to the liver, especially in chronic conditions. It is used extensively to decongest the liver due to blood conditions or excesses. It is also helpful in hepatitis, cholecystitis, heaviness in the eyes, muscle cramping and musculo-tendon tension anywhere in the body.

BL 19 – Gall Bladder Shu Point – 1.5 cun lateral to the lower border of the spinous process of **T10**

This acupoint is useful in treating gall bladder and liver imbalance. Symptoms would include cholecystitis, nausea, bitter taste, jaundice and shoulder pain. Used also as a local point in thoracic pain, spasm and scoliosis (as are all the thoracic bladder points)

BL 20 – Spleen Shu Point – 1.5 cun lateral to the lower border of the spinous border of **T11**

This acupoint is used widely in all cases of spleen energy deficiency. Symptoms include chronic tiredness and weariness, weakness of the limbs, sweating, flaccidity, water retention, tendency to gain weight, abdominal distension, loose stools, some gynaecological conditions.

BL 21 – Stomach Shu Point – 1.5 cun lateral to the lower border of **T12**

This acupoint is widely used in stomach related condition. These include gastritis, stomach distension, indigestion, poor appetite, abdominal distension and diarrhoea.

BL 22 – Triple Energizer (Sanjiao) Shu Point – 1.5 lateral to the lower border of the spinous process of **L1**

This acupoint is important in resolving dampness, opening the water passages and promoting urination. It is used in water retention, urinary disorders, swelling and oedema of the abdomen and limbs. Moxabustion and Cupping are useful on this point in these chronic conditions.

BL23 – Kidney Shu Point – 1.5 cun lateral to the lower border of the spinous process of **L2**

This acupoint is used to tonify the kidney energy. It is a major point for many disorders of the lumbo-sacral spine, pelvis and legs. Symptoms include lumbar pain and weakness, low back pain, chronic weakness or paralysis of the legs, coldness in the lower back and loins, sciatica and restless legs. It may also be used as an adjunct point in treating chronic urinary conditions. It remains one of the most important acupoints that deals with lethargy and chronic tiredness. It is an excellent self-help acupressure point alongside adjacent points in helping lumbar fibrositis by vigorously massaging the area with clenched fists several times a day.

BL 25 – Large intestine Shu Point – 1.5 cun lateral to the lower border of the spinous process of **L4**

This acupoint is a major player in the treatment of many large bowel conditions including constipation and diarrhoea, ileo-caecal valve syndrome, abdominal rumbling, pain and distension. It is also useful, alongside other local points, in helping low back pain, sciatica and spasm.

BL27 – Small Intestine Shu Point – 1.5 cun lateral to the posterior midline, level with the **first sacral foramen.**

This acupoint is used extensively in both small bowel imbalance and urinary conditions. Symptoms include intestinal pain, enteritis, difficulty in urination, incontinence, sacral pain, sacroiliitis and sciatica.

BL 28 – Bladder Shu Point – 1.5 lateral to the midline at the level of the **second sacral foramen**

This acupoint is influential in treating bladder conditions. Symptoms include urine incontinence, urinary tract discomfort and cystitis, plus impotence and genital pain.

The Outer Bladder Line

The Outer Bladder Line is part of the bladder meridian that run roughly parallel to the spine, 3 cun (four fingers width) lateral to the spine and 1.5 cun (two fingers width) lateral to the inner bladder line. The clear majority, but not all, of the Inner Line Back Transporting points has an 'equivalent' point on the Outer Line. This important line of acupoints are the least understood in the whole of acupuncture as to their purpose and indications. Tradition dictates that each one is the 'emotional equivalent' of its Inner channel partner, and you would not be far wrong from this assumption. Some of them are related to the important spinal chakras as well as to endocrine glands via the sympathetic nervous system. Figure 1.5.6 gives a diagrammatic representation of these points.

BL 42 – Door of the Soul – 3 cun lateral to the spinous process of **T3 level with BL 13**

This acupoint has similar properties as its Inner Bladder Line companion – BL 13 in that it is used in many respiratory conditions. Its main use though is in helping the emotions associated with the Lung and Metal element. These are sadness, grief, melancholy and some aspects of depression associated with grief.

BL43 – Vital Region – 3 cun lateral to the spinous process of **T4 level with BL 14**

This acupoint is used extensively in many respiratory conditions including chronic cough, shortness of breath, asthma, and bronchitis, even though it is linked with the pericardium. Its main claim to fame is that it helps boost energy in chronic disease. Either tonifying acupuncture or stimulating acupressure are required. If patients have chronic respiratory, cardiac or throat conditions, treatment on this point will help boost their vital force. I have used this point successfully in treating patients who were desperately ill. It is a better point than ST 36 in these situations. Practitioners of the manipulative and soft tissue arts appreciate the value of mobilising the fourth vertebra in chronic spinal and internal organic conditions to enable them to gain more energy. It can be used in isolation or in tandem with both BL 13 and BL 14.

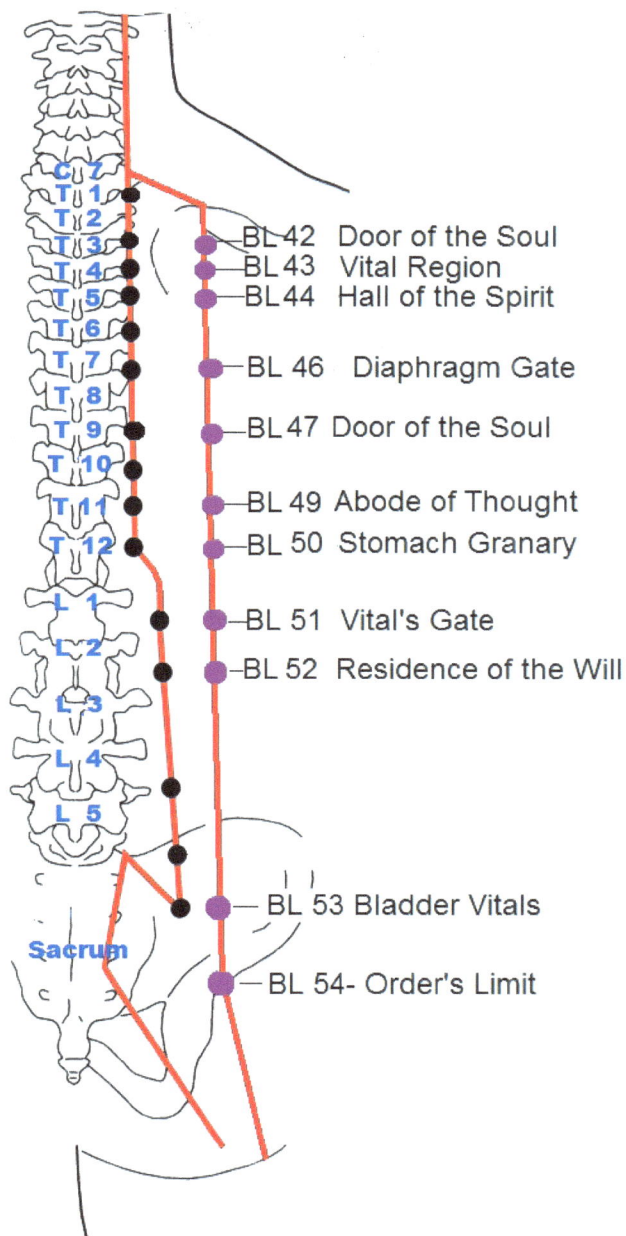

Figure 1.5.6. The Outer Bladder Line

BL 44 – Hall of the Spirit – 3 cun lateral to the spinous process of **T5 level with BL 15**

This acupoint is excellent in the treatment of many psychosomatic conditions including restlessness, anxiety, nightmares, panic attacks, insomnia, some forms of epilepsy and stress in general. It is also used to treat cardiac conditions alongside BL 15. In esoteric medicine this acupoint is associated with the posterior Heart chakra, that deals with many emotional conditions. In children under the age of seven, this point also relates to the thymus gland. Also, used in the treatment of idiopathic scoliosis.

BL 46 – Diaphragm Gate – 3 cun lateral to the spinous process of **T7 level with BL 17**

This acupoint works in union with BL 17 in the treatment of blood related conditions. It is also associated with the treatment of stress and indigestion and dyspepsia due to anxiety and worry. Also, used in the treatment of idiopathic scoliosis.

BL 47 – Door of the Soul – 3 cun lateral to the spinous process of **T9 level with BL 18**

This acupoint is used extensively with BL 18 in the treatment of liver energy imbalance. Emotional symptoms are those associated with the liver and the Wood element, namely anger, rage, irritability, frustration, anxiety boredom and lack of will. Also, used in idiopathic scoliosis.

BL 49 – Abode of Thought – 3 cun lateral to the spinous process of **T11 level with BL 20**

This acupoint is very influential in treating physical and emotional conditions associated with the spleen and stomach. Physical symptoms include abdominal distension, nausea, vomiting, jaundice, indigestion and some symptoms of diabetes. Emotional symptoms include depression, worry, poor concentration, diminishing memory and with people who do much thinking and pondering e.g. making decisions. Also, used in the treatment of idiopathic scoliosis.

BL 50 – Stomach Granary – 3 cun lateral to the spinous process of **T12 level with BL 21**

This acupoint is used to harmonise the stomach and benefit digestion – used in conjunction with both BL 21 and BL 50 (above). Used extensively in depression, worry and poor concentration.

BL 51 – Vital's Gate – 3 cun lateral to the spinous process of **L1 level with BL 22**

 This acupoint is used in conjunction with BL 22 in treating dampness and urinary conditions. It is excellent for frequent urination (weak bladder) and in some cases of bed wetting (enuresis) PS. In child enuresis, the best acupoint is a non-meridian point called Yi Niao Xue, situated on the sole of the foot in the middle of the fifth metatarso-phalangeal crease. Also, a useful point on the same point on the palm of the hand by the little finger.

BL 52 – Residence of the Will – 3 cun lateral to the spinous process of **L2 level with BL 23**

As with all Outer Bladder points, BL 52 has both physical and emotional properties. It helps urination and strengthens the lumbar region as well as aiding BL 23 in treating kidney symptoms. Its emotional properties are paramount, however, in that it helps the patient deal with situations of fear, anxiety and lack of will power. If the will is at a low ebb this point will help strengthen the resolve (once the cause is known).

BL 53 – Bladder Vitals – 3 cun lateral to the spinous process of **S2 level with BL 28**

This acupoint is used in low back pain, sciatica, gluteal pain and sacro-iliac conditions, with BL 28 and BL 32. It has few other uses.

BL 54 – Order's Limit – 3 cun lateral to the midline at the level of the **4ᵗʰ sacral foramen**

This acupoint is at the highest part of the buttock, so either a long needle or very firm acupressure is required here. It is very useful in sports therapy, using the knuckle, in the treatment of localised pain, sciatica, piriformis and gluteal pain and spasm. It is also used in constipation and lymphatic obstruction.

The Sacral Points

The acupoints BL 27 to BL 35 are all located around the sacrum. Figure 1.5.7 refers

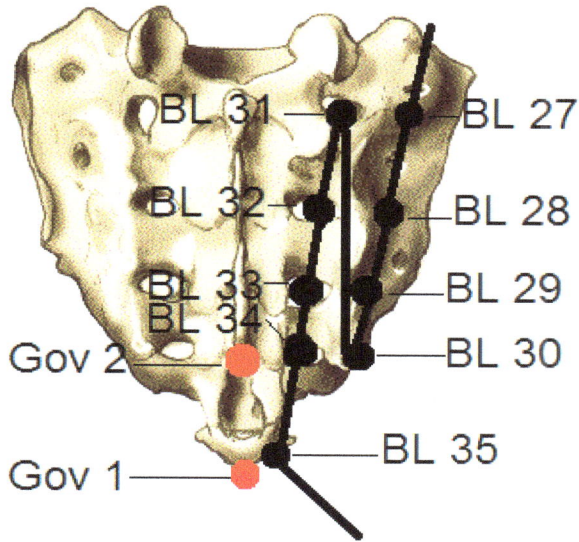

Figure 1.5.7 The Sacral Bladder Points

BL 27 and BL28 have been previously described as the Small Intestine and Bladder Back Transporting Points.

BL 29 – Middle Spine Shu –1.5 cun lateral to the midline at the level of the 3rd **sacral foramen**

BL 30 – White Ring Shu – 1.5 cun lateral to the midline at the level of the 4th **sacral foramen**

BL 31 – Upper Bone Hole – over the 1st sacral foramen

BL 32 – Second Bone Hole – over the 2nd sacral foramen

BL33 – Middle Bone Hole – over the 3rd sacral foramen

BL 34 - Lower Bone Hole – over the 4th sacral foramen

BL 35 – Meeting of Yang – level with the tip of the coccyx just adjacent to BL 1

These seven acupoints may be described together as, in practice, they are often used in treatment together. Symptoms include lumbo-sacral pain and stiffness, sciatica, irregular menstruation, vaginal prolapse, impotence and difficulty with urination. All the points answer very well to massage and other body work in all cases of sluggishness of the gluteal and piriformis muscles, chronic conditions of the kidneys and bladder, uterus, testes, sacrum and coccyx. One of the very best ways to treat these points (and this area in general) is with Connective Tissue Massage (CTM). This is a stimulating type of massage that uses the medial aspect of the middle finger, with or without oil, in deep and controlled strokes. These acupoints and this technique should *not* be performed in pregnancy.

Small Intestine Meridian

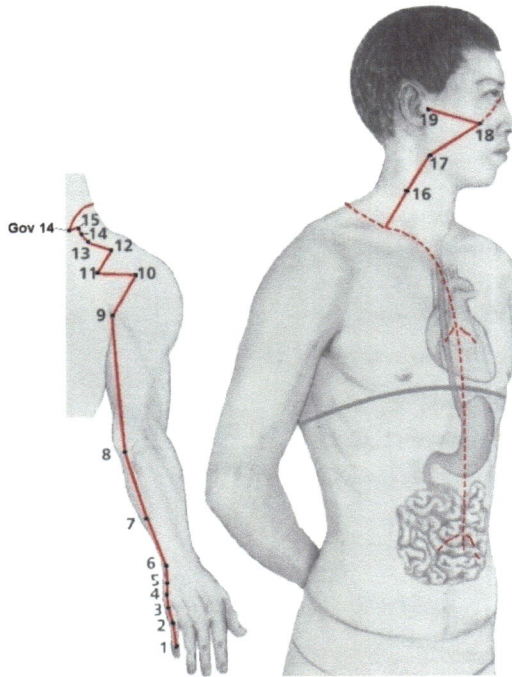

Figure 1.5.8 Small Intestine Meridian

The Small Intestine meridian is one of the Yang aspects of the Fire Element and consists of 19 acupoints, commencing at the lateral nail point on the little finger, travelling up the posterior lateral aspect of the forearm, posterior aspect of the upper arm, where it zigzags over the scapula and at SI 15 connects to Gov 14 (C7-T1), before returning to the anterior aspect of the neck. The surface channel then ascends to the outer aspect of the face and ends at the front of the ear. An inner pathway descends from Gov 14 to the heart and small intestine. The four most important acupoints regarding the spine are SI 13,14, 15 and SI 3.

SI 13 – Crooked Wall – at the medial end of the **suprascapular fossa** in the trapezius muscle.

SI 14 – Outer Shoulder Point – 3 cun lateral to the **spinous process of T1**

SI 15 – Middle Shoulder Point – 2 cun lateral to the lower border of C7 (Gov 14) at the end of the **transverse process of T1**

These acupoints may be considered as the most superior (anatomically speaking) of the Inner Bladder line in that they are just to the side of the spine and have a similar action. A deep channel goes from SI 15 this point to Gov 14, then on to the heart and small intestine. These points may be used together in deep massage affecting the upper fibres of trapezius and the underlying muscles. They are very useful in headaches, migraine and tension in the occiput and head.

SI 3 – Back Stream – located at the proximal end of the **5th metacarpal** bone on the ulnar surface. This acupoint is far and away the most influential on this channel and has a great influence on the spine. It is used in pain on the outer aspect of the face, shoulders and neck. Its very special property, though, is that it is the Key (Opening) point of the Governor (Du Mai) meridian. It may be used with acupuncture or pressure in the treatment of most spinal pain – especially the cervical region and remains one of our best points in self-help for pain in this region. It is linked with BL 62 by the ankle – this will be dealt with in the practical part of Book Two.

Large Intestine Meridian

The Large Intestine meridian is the Yang aspect of the Metal Element and consists of 20 points on its surface channel. As illustration 1.5.9 shows it commences at the index finger, travels up the forearm and back of the upper arm, over the shoulder, joins the spine at Gov 14 before it travels up the neck and ends by the nose. Internal pathways travel from the spine to the large bowel and lungs and from the neck to the mouth. There are 3 extremely important acupoints on this meridian – LI 4, LI 15 and the junction with the lower cervical spine from LI 16.

LI 4 – Joining Valley (Hegu) – located on the dorsum of the hand to the side of the mid-point of the second metacarpal bone in **the first interosseous muscle.** This acupoint is probably the most used in the entire body due to its indications in the treatment of multiple syndromes. It is colloquially called 'the great eliminator' and, as such, is used to eliminate pain and discomfort especially around the upper spine, shoulder and head, although it may be used in pain relief anywhere. It also has a great affinity for bowel imbalance as it is the 'source' point of the large intestine. Do not use this point in pregnancy.

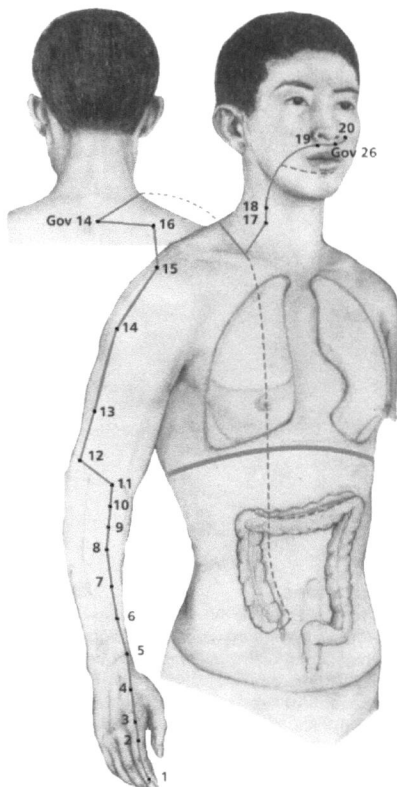

Figure 1.5.9 The Large Intestine Meridian

LI 15 – Shoulder Bone – located at the lateral aspect of the shoulder at the level of the **acromio-clavicular joint** in the large hollow when the arm is abducted. This acupoint has a powerful action on upper spine and shoulder pain and discomfort. It is also the physical acupoint of the Shoulder chakra that is associated with the Throat chakra at both Con 22 and Gov 14.

LI 16 – LI 17 via Gov 14. A deep channel passes from LI 16 to Gov 14 at C7-T1 before proceeding to LI 17 at the neck. This deep channel is very important in highlighting the importance of Gov 14 (posterior Throat chakra) and its affinity for the shoulder and the bowel.

Gall Bladder Meridian

The Gall Bladder meridian represents the Yang aspect of the Wood element. The surface Gall Bladder channel contains 44 points commencing at the eye and ending on the 4th toe. It has a most unusual journey – probably *the* most convoluted of all the meridians. It links the Bladder, Stomach, Liver, Small Intestine and Governor channels along its course. It is the only channel to appear on the lateral side of the body. Figure 1.5.10 refers.

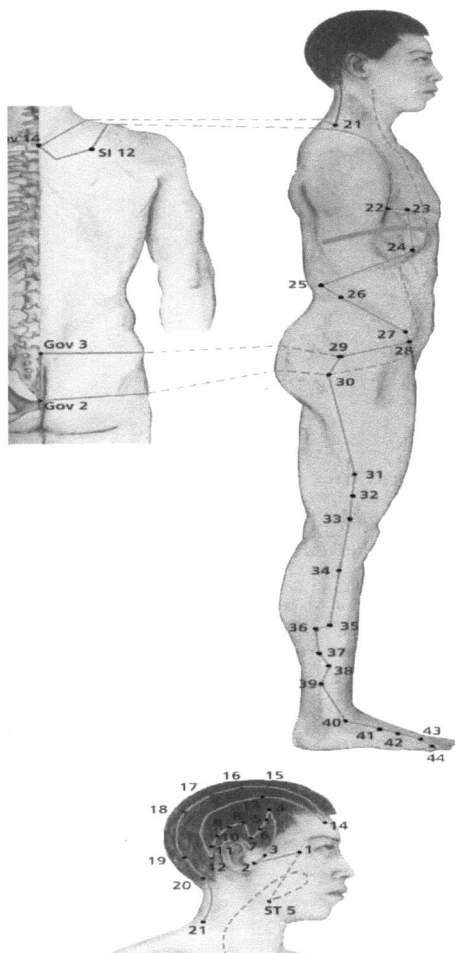

Figure 1.5.10 The Gall Bladder meridian

As the illustration shows, the meridian has contact with the spine at two separate areas, the cervical and the lumbar spine.

GB 21 -GB 22 via Gov 14 The deep channel between these two acupoints travels to our old friend Gov 14 at the C7-T1 level and to SI 12. The lower Gall Bladder points therefore have an influence on the cervical spine as well as the shoulder.

GB 29 and GB 30 via the Governor channel between Gov 3 and Gov 2. GB 29 and GB 30 are the only acupoints that locally effect on the hip joint, although many other points have an influence. A deep channel travels directly to the spine between L4-5 and the sacro-coccyx junction. This explains the affinity that the sacral and lower bladder points have for the hip.

That completes the 'anatomy' of the meridians and acupoints that pass through or have influence on the spine.

The Governor meridian, Inner and Outer Bladder Line acupoints and their influence on the autonomic nervous system

The autonomic nervous system and its relationship with the spine was discussed in Part One. There is little doubt that acupuncture/acupressure and many other physical therapies work through the integration of the autonomic nervous system (ANS) with the central nervous system (CNS). Acupuncture has utilised the Back-Supporting Points on the Inner Bladder and Outer Bladder Lines for centuries, with no clear rationale as to their viability. Other disciplines such as some aspects of osteopathy and chiropractic also promulgate the vitalism approach of energy medicine by purporting to effect internal organs, endocrine glands, lymphatic flow etc. by the mobilising of the vertebrae or adjustments of the facet joints. Below – Figure 1.5.11 - is an illustration that shows the interaction of the Governor meridian and the Inner and Outer Line acupoints of the Bladder meridian with the sympathetic and parasympathetic nervous system. Please note that this is purely diagrammatic in that the paravertebral sympathetic chain is much closer to the spine i.e. over the transverse processes, but for clarity and to show the interrelationship of the two sections of the Bladder meridian, it was shown outside the spinal region and being directly influenced by the outer Bladder line. The diagram shows that internal organs may be influenced by therapeutic disciplines on the spine. These would include the following: -

- Manipulation by any means (chiropractic, osteopathic etc.) that realigns the vertebra or eases undue spasm or tension in the intrinsic muscles that have caused facet joint locking (fixation).
- Acupuncture, either by locally placed needles or needles at a distance may have the same effect as manipulation
- Localised acupressure has the same effect as acupuncture
- Reflexology, either by itself or in tandem with acupressure may have the same affect.
- Deep massage on the area may also ease tension in the sympathetic nerve supply to ease organ tension
- Touch therapy using the posterior major chakras will have the same action
- It is possible that non-contact and distance healing also has the same affect, especially if you consider, as I do, that 'all is energy'. Examples of this would be radionics or distance healing via radiesthesia or 'projected thought'. See my book on Distance Analysis and Healing for details.

Vagus Nerve

Medulla

Gov 16 — Occiput — Superior Cervical Ganglion

Eye — From III

Gov 15 — C 1

Lacrimal Gland, Nose, Palate — From VII

Submandibular Gland Sublingual Gland — From VII

Mouth, Parotid Gland — From IX

Cranial Nerve Supply

C 4
C 5
C 6
C 7

Middle Cervical Ganglion

Inferior Cervical Ganglion

Gov 14 — T 1 — BL 11
Gov 13 — T 2

Larynx - Trachea

Lung

Heart

BL 13 — BL 42

Gov 12 — T 3
T 4 — BL 14 — BL 43

Greater Splanchnic Nerve — Celiac Plexus

Oesophagus

Stomach

T 5 — BL 15 — BL 44

Abdominal Blood Vessels

Gov 11 — T 6 — BL 16

Gov 10 — T 7 — BL 17 — BL 46

Lesser Splanchnic Nerve

Gov 9 — T 8 — BL 47

T 9 — BL 18

Gov 8 — T 10 — BL 19

Superior Mesenteric Plexus

Liver

Gall Bladder

Gov 7 — T 11 — BL 20 — BL 49

Spleen

Pancreas

Gov 6 — T 12 — BL 21 — BL 50

Suprarenal

Kidney

L 1 — BL 51

Gov 5 — BL 22

Inferior Mesenteric Plexus

Large Intestine

L 2 — BL 23 — BL 52

Small Intestine

Gov 4 — L 3 — BL 24

L 4 — BL 25

Paravertebral Sympathetic Chain

Rectum

Gov 3 — L 5 — BL 26

Bladder

Testes/Uterus

BL 27

SACRUM — BL 28 — BL 53

Pelvic Splanchnic Nerves

BL 54

Gov 2 — Coccyx

Sympathetic Nerves ——
Parasympathetic Nerves ——
CNS Nerve Roots ——

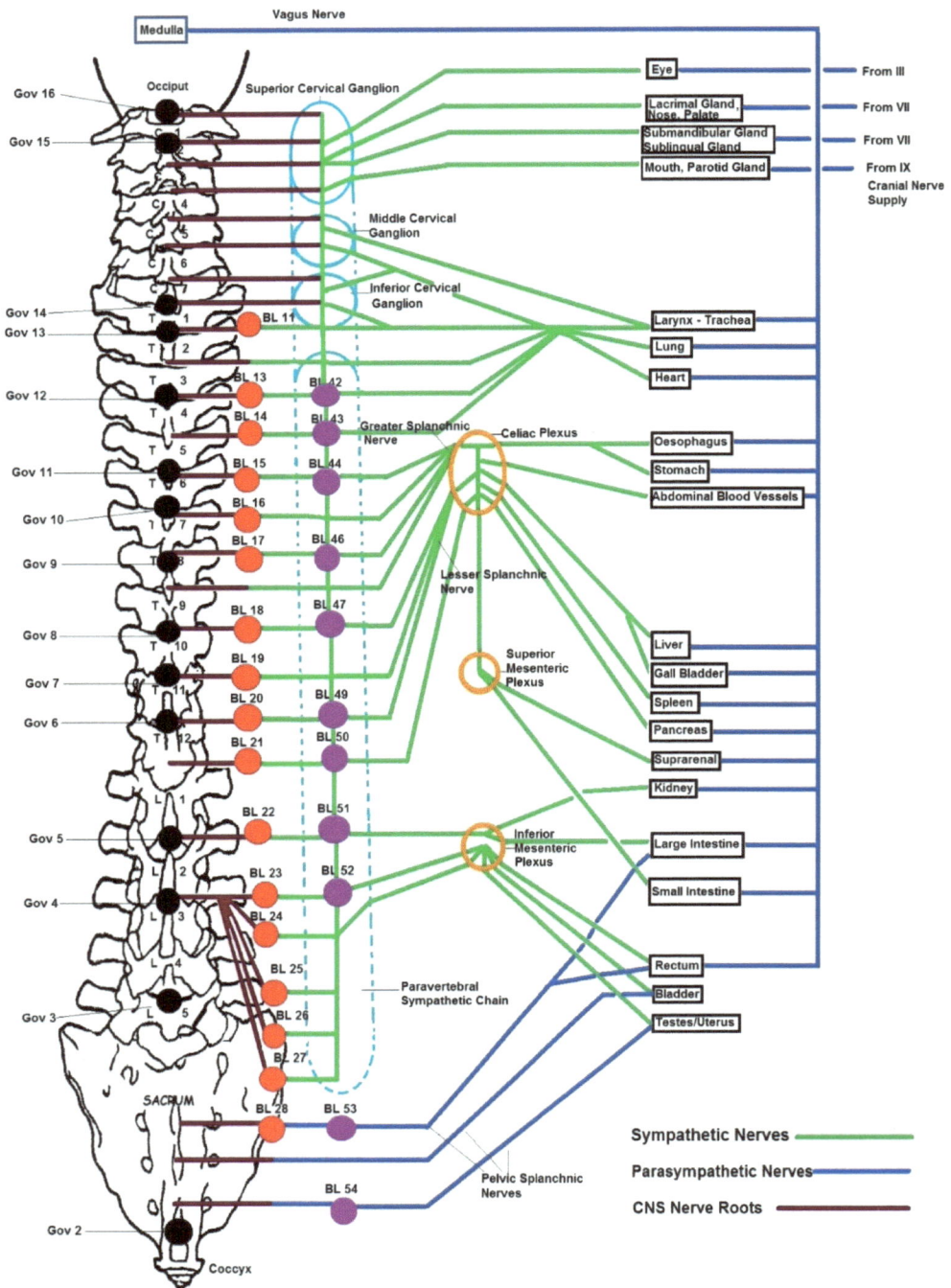

JRC copyright 2016

Figure 1.5.11 Diagrammatic Representation of the Relationship of the Spine, Governor, Inner Bladder and Outer Bladder Acupoints with the Autonomic Nervous System – replicated in Book Two

Trigger Points

The treatment of non-acupuncture trigger points has become very popular in the last twenty years with the rise in popularity of western (medical) acupuncture where the relief of pain is paramount. The phrase 'trigger points' was first coined by Dr. Janet Travell in 1942 describing a pain that could not be explained by findings in a neurological examination. The inside of the body is covered with soft tissue called fascia, that covers evert structure including organs, muscles, nerves and blood vessels. The fascia that covers muscles is call myofascia. When the myofascia is stressed from overuse or trauma it can tear and adhere together. These adhesions are called "trigger points" and can prevent the muscles from working well. Trigger points lead to an increase in muscle stiffness and tenderness and a decrease in range-of-motion. The discomfort from trigger points can radiate from the adhesion (referred pain). Trigger points in muscles may also be called fibrositic nodules, that leads to fibrositis. The clear majority of trigger points lie in myofascia. A trigger point, of course, may also be any acute painful spot on the skin that is a referral from somewhere else. Examples of this type would be *Erbs* point and *Klumpkes* point that are acute sites on the trapezius muscle caused by conditions (usually spondylosis) of C5-6 and C7-T1 respectively. The trigger points in the myofascia of muscles that are directly connected with the spine are discussed in the next chapter and their treatment in Book Two. Figure 1.5.12 shows some of the anterior muscles with their trigger points positions

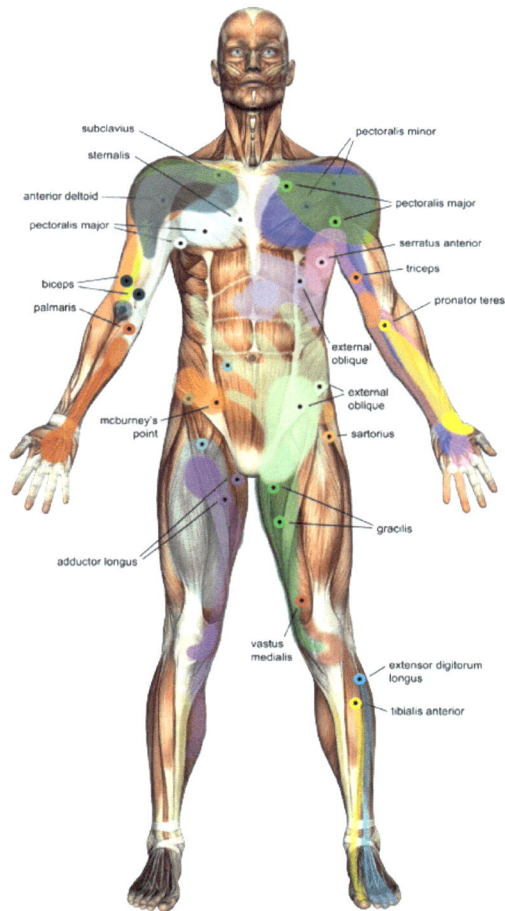

Figure 1.5.12 Trigger Points of Anterior Muscles

Chapter Six – The Energetic Muscles of the Spine

This chapter will describe some of the important muscles that act over and move the spine, not only anatomically but their energetic and holistic influence. It is impossible to describe every muscle here so I have chosen the salient ones. The energetic part of the equation is taken from the following sources: -

- Applied Kinesiology (AK)

- Trigger Points according to Travell and Simons

- Traditional Chinese medicine (TCM)

TCM tells us that all muscles of the body are associated with the **Liver** energy and the fascia, tendons and cartilage that support the muscles are associated with the **Spleen and Stomach** energies. Some authorities state that muscles are linked with the Spleen and just tendons with the Liver, but in practical terms of using this information for many years, I cannot agree. Individual muscles may be associated with other internal organic energy systems. Practical applications of these will be in Book Two.

Cervical Spine Muscles

Muscles that flex the head and neck

1. Longus Colli

2. Longus Capitis

3. Rectus Capitis Anterior

4. Sternocleidomastoid

5. Scalenus Anterior

Longus Colli, Longus Capitis and Rectus Capitis Anterior – (Figure 1.6.1)
Origin - Insertion – Action They represent the deepest of the anterior neck muscles. They flex the head when acting together and side flex the head on the neck individually. See diagram for the various attachments.
Nerve Supply - The nerve supply to these muscles range between C1-2 and C4-5 depending on which insertion is innervated.
Trigger Points - When these muscles are feeling pressurised due to postural changes to the individual vertebrae that they act over, the trigger points may be felt on the lateral aspect of the transverse process. Beyond that, these deep muscles are very difficult to locate or palpate.
Holistic Considerations AK tells us that they are related to Stomach energy. This is because the Stomach meridian energy line passes through the region. In TCM, the stomach's energy links are the mouth, taste, and food absorption. It is part of the Earth Element (with the Spleen) and its emotional role is in worry and depression. So, when muscles that are linked with the stomach are in spasm or pain for no reason, it could be caused by poor nourishment, worry/depression or that we are not grounded in our thoughts and actions. The latter is typical of the emotional aetiology of upper cervical imbalance.

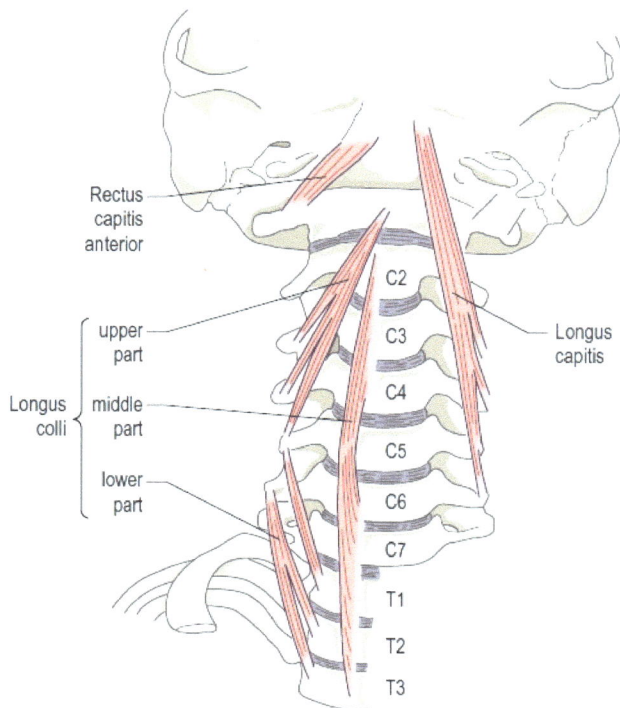

Figure 1.6.1 Rectus Capitis, Longus Colli and Longus Capitis muscles

Sternocleidomastoid (SCM) – (Figure 1.6.2)

Origin - Insertion - Action This muscle, often abbreviated to just sternomastoid, has a common proximal insertion on mastoid process of the temporal bone and two distal insertions on the manubrium of the sternum and the clavicle. Unilateral contraction laterally flexes the head on the neck, rotating it to the opposite side and side flexes the neck. When both muscles work together they draw the head forwards and help in elevating the thorax.

Nerve Supply – The motor supply of the SCM is by the spinal part of the Accessory Nerve (XI Cranial) and the sensory supply is from C2-3

Trigger Points – There are several trigger points along the length of the SCM. These may cause neck pain, blurred vision, headache (mostly over the eye), migraine, eye symptoms such as drooping of the eyelid, ear symptoms such as hearing loss and tinnitus, also sinusitis. This is a very important and influential muscle. Treatment in Part Four

Holistic Considerations – Spasm of the SCM causes torticollis (wry neck) and can cause considerable deviation to the atlas and axis when is spasm. AK tells us that it is associated with the Stomach energy (see above for description) and wry neck or associated symptoms may be caused by some food intolerances as well as stress of modern living. Do not assume that all so called mechanical conditions have a mechanical cause – they don't!

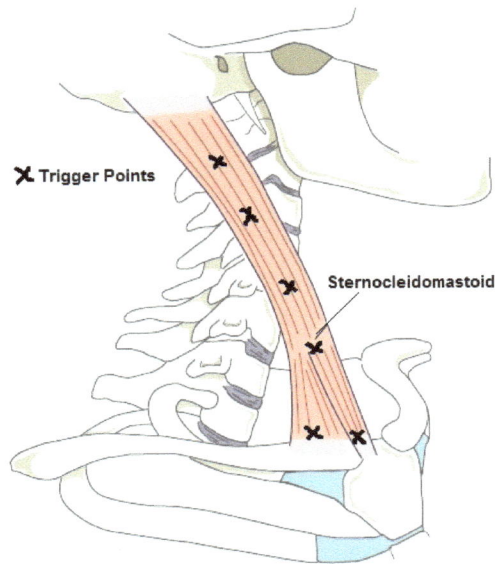

Figure 1.6.2 Sternocleidomastoid muscle

<u>Muscles that side flex the head and neck</u>
1. Scalenus Anterior, Scalenus Posterior and Scalenus Medius

2. Levator Scapulae

3. Sternocleidomastoid

4. Splenius Capitis

Scalenus Anterior, Scalenus Posterior and Scalenus Medius (Figure 1.6.3)

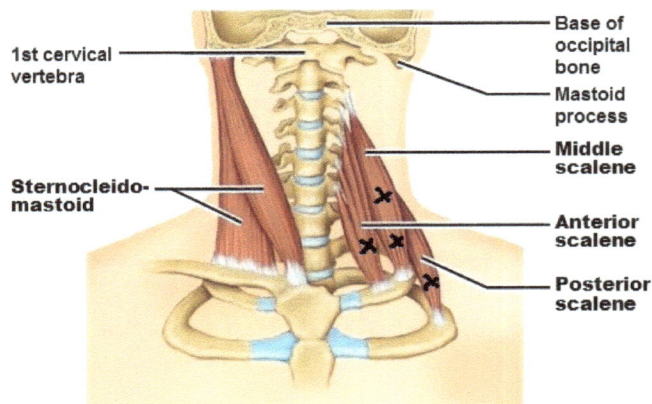

Figure 1.6.3 The Scalene Muscles

The Scalene muscles are usually grouped together as they can be considered as three parts of the same muscle.

<u>Origin – Insertion – Action</u> They arise from the transverse processes of C2-C6 and Scalenus Anterior and Medius attach to the top of the first rib whilst Scalenus Posterior attaches to the second rib. They have two actions – they elevate the first two ribs, thus aiding inspiration, and the flex and side flex the cervical spine.

68

Nerve Supply – Scalenus Anterior is innervated from C4,5 and 6 – Scalenus Medius from C3,4,5,6,7 and Scalenus Posterior from C6,7,8

Trigger Points – there are several trigger points commonly found on these muscles (see diagram) that may cause pain and paraesthesia in the arm. If these muscles go into spasm they can affect the section of the brachial plexus that passes between the muscular insertions on the ribs (C4,5,6 nerve root)

Holistic Considerations – as they are grouped with other neck flexors, they are associated with Stomach energy (see description above). These muscles are also affected in respiratory conditions (e.g. asthma) where breathing is limited. Tightness and congestion in these muscles may cause a condition called Thoracic Outlet Syndrome. They are also involved when the person is unfortunate enough to have a cervical rib and spasm may cause an elevated first rib.

Levator Scapulae (Figure 1.6.4)

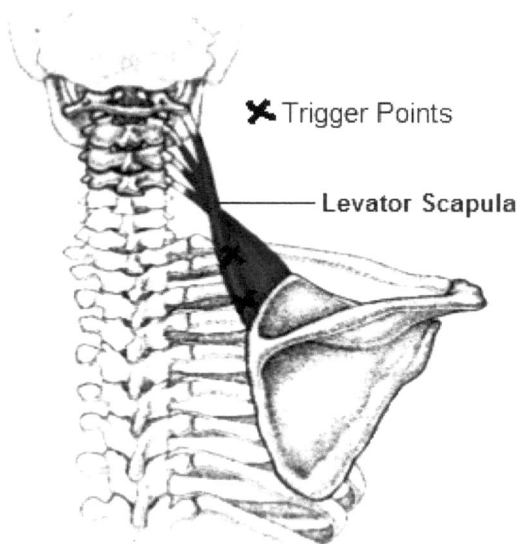

Figure 1.6.4 Levator Scapulae muscle

Origin – Insertion – Action – This muscle lies deep to the SCM in its upper part and deep to the trapezius in the lower part. It attaches to the transverse processes of C1, 2, 3 and 4 and inserts on the medial border of the scapula. Note how its tendons twist around at its origin. Working with the trapezius it helps stabilize the scapula during arm movements and it also rotates the scapula as well as side flexing the neck. Due to its twisting tendons, it also extends the neck when both muscles are working.

Nerve Supply – Innervated by C3,4 and 5

Trigger Points – There may be two trigger points on this muscle, but they are very common. The lower one near to the scapula insertion is also called 'Erbs' Point which is a trigger point arising from C5-6 nerve root inflammation. Pain from this point is therefore directed down the arm following the course of the radial nerve.

Holistic Considerations – Once again it is associated with the Stomach energy. Pain and spasm in this muscle due to either a mechanical trauma or emotional stress may give rise to tension in the throat and the thyroid gland, causing thyroid imbalance.

Splenius Capitis (Figure 1.6.5)

Origin – Insertion – Action – This muscle lies deep to the SCM and trapezius. It originates from the spinous processes of C6, 7, T1-4 and inserts below the lateral third of the nuchal line and the mastoid process of the temporal bone. Unilateral contraction produces extension, side flexion and rotation of the neck and head and contraction of both muscles extends the head and neck.

Nerve Supply – Innervated from C3,4 and 5

Trigger Point – just one on this muscle, but very important. It lies on the nuchal line and is better known as acupuncture point GB 12. When inflamed, this give pain over the top of the head and eyes.

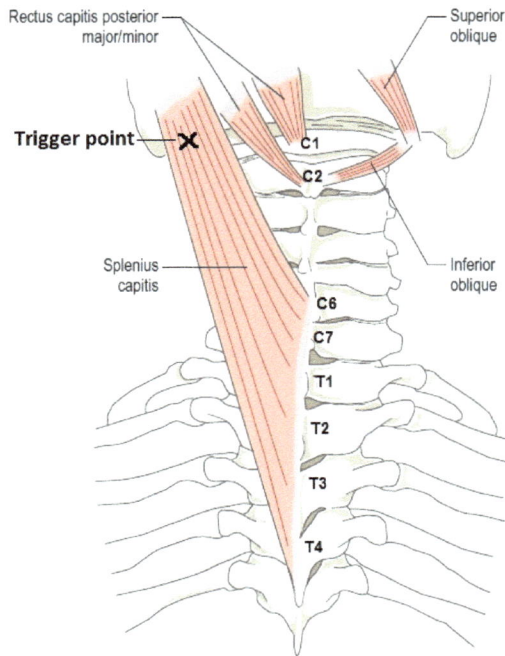

Figure 1.6.5 Splenius Capitis, Rectus Capitis Posteriors and Oblique muscles

Holistic Considerations – Once again, related with stomach energy. The trigger point, though, is on the gall bladder meridian so spasm in this muscle can give rise to gall bladder imbalance (and vice versa)

Muscles that extend the head and neck

1. Levator Scapulae

2. Trapezius

3. Splenius Capitis

4. The Suboccipital Muscles

5. Erector Spinae

Trapezius (Figure 1.6.6)

Origin – Insertion – Action It is the largest and most superficial muscle in the region and the most powerful. It is a large, flat, triangular muscle that forms a trapezoid when looked at as two muscles. It originates on the occiput, the ligamentum nuchae and the spinous processes of C7 down to T12. It inserts on the clavicle plus the acromion and spine of the scapula. Its fibres are roughly divided into three sections. The upper fibres elevate and rotate the scapula and shoulder; the middle fibres adduct the scapula and the lower

fibres pull the scapula downwards. Working together, all the groups pull the shoulder blade backwards towards the spine (retraction). The illustration shows just two sections as this is more commonplace.
Nerve Supply – The motor supply is from the Accessory Nerve (XI cranial) and the sensory input is from C3,4

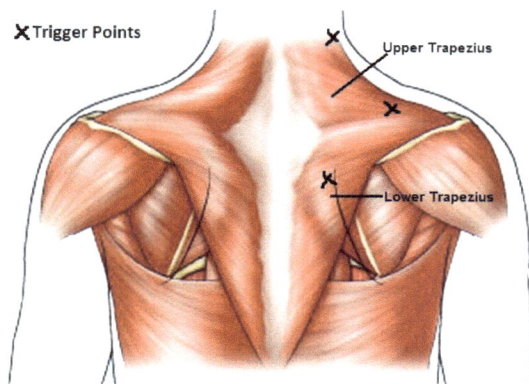

Figure 1.6.6 Trapezius muscle

Trigger Points – This muscle is prone to spasm, tension and trigger points and are a common cause of direct and referred pain. Pain and spasm in this muscle has proliferated due to the lifestyles and work mode of people – mostly caused by staring at computer screens all day. The most common trigger points are shown. There is a very common one that relates to GB 12 on the lower end of the occiput that gives pain to the side of the face. This is the same as the Splenius Capitis trigger point (the trapezius overlaps this muscle). Another common site is between the neck and shoulder between GB 21 and SI 15. This gives referred pain down the arm towards the thumb. A lesser trigger point is found to the side of the spine around the T2 level. This also gives pain down the arm but the ulnar side this time – also some burning pain around the shoulder blade.
Holistic Considerations – AK states that the trapezius is related to the Spleen meridian. This shows a slight departure from all the other neck muscles being affiliated with the Stomach, but it is still within the Earth Element. The muscle may be affected from its many attachments – it is prone to pain/spasm from the occipital and lower cervical attachments that gives referred pain to the head and shoulders, and from the T12 attachment where tension in that region may affect the rest of the muscle. Due to its relationship with the Spleen, with continuous spasm there are often auto-immune symptoms such as sore throats, infections and anaemia. Its nerve supply (XI Cranial) is also significant and practical remedies for imbalance will be discussed in Book Two.

The Suboccipital muscles – Rectus Capitis Posterior Major: Rectus Capitis Posterior Minor: Obliquus Capitis Superior and Obliquus Capitis Inferior (Figure 1.6.5)
Origin – Insertion – Action – These four tiny muscles form the group known as the suboccipital muscles. The Rectus Capitis Posterior Major muscle originates on the spinous process of the Axis (C2) vertebra and inserts at the lateral part of the inferior nuchal line on the occiput. The Minor muscle originates distally to the tubercle on the arch of the Atlas (C1) and inserts to the medial part on the nuchal line of the occiput. The Obliquus Capitis Superior is attached to the transverse process of the Atlas and inserts on the nuchal line of the occiput. The Obliquus Capitis Inferior is the largest of the subocciptals and is attached to both transverse processes of the Atlas and Axis. They are tiny muscles but they 'pack a punch' as they are all

important in stabilizing the occipito-atlas (C0-1) junction. This junction is also referred to as the cranial base.

Nerve Supply – They are all innervated from C0-1

Trigger Points – Although these small muscles rarely have trigger points per se, when the atlas, axis or cranial base is affected by trauma or stress, the insertions on the transverse processes become very tender, often giving referred pain to the forehead, top of head, eyes and affecting the arterial flow within the area. Migraine is a common result of imbalance to these muscles.

Holistic Considerations – The Minor muscle is connected to the spinal dura, thus affecting the cerebrospinal fluid flow when it is in a state of tension. All the suboccipital muscles are related to the Stomach meridian energy flow. As they are important in stabilizing the occiput, they may be affected, not only by local postural changes but by changes to the sacrum (which is related to the occiput – details elsewhere). Thus, constant tension in the suboccipital muscles may give rise to lower back pain, sacral instability and hamstring shortening – and vice versa (as above – so below). The Rectus Capitis muscles are involved in trigeminal nerve conditions that affect the cervical spine and head. Practical details give in Book Two

Thoracic Spine Muscles

There are scores of small and long muscles that are attached to the thoracic spinal complex. The small muscles include the Multifidus, Rotatores, Interspinales and the Intertransversarii. They are all very important in giving stability to the mid-section of the spine as well as the rib cage. The only three muscles that need be mentioned in detail are the Erector Spinae, Latissimus Dorsi and the Diaphragm.

Erector Spinae (Figure 1.6.7)

This large and powerful muscles (sometimes called 'Sacrospinalis') is a complex muscle that may be divided into three columns – the Iliocostalis, Longissimus and Spinalis.

Origin – Insertion - Action The muscle has influence over the whole spine as it arises from the deep lumbo-sacral fascia and inserts in the cervical spine. If you count the neck extensors as being part of this huge muscle (as some authorities do) then the insertion is at the base of the occiput bone. Each section of the muscle has both a local action and a large axial action depending on the insertion. The main action of this muscle is to extend the spine but also to maintain stability on the part at which it inserts.

Nerve Supply It has an extensive nerve supply, depending on the site of the muscle

Trigger Points These may be various and extensive depending on which part of the muscle is in spasm or affected by internal or external trauma. I have indicated one major trigger point at app. the lateral aspect of T6-7. This is very common in all manner of spinal conditions and pain. This often gives rise to internal discomfort around the solar plexus and diaphragm. It also gives rise to pain and further spasm up and down the spine, giving further symptoms where weakness occurs. This part of the spine is prone to being 'weak' as it is the very central part of the whole spine and is subject to many external and internal forces.

Holistic Considerations. In AK, the internal organ/energy link is the Bladder meridian. This makes a lot of sense as the Bladder meridian lies parallel to the spine and affects the whole of the muscle from the cervical to sacral region. Imbalance in this muscle may occur because of trauma and accident, arthritic changes and poor posture as well as influence from the legs and arms that may put extra strain on the muscle. The Erector Spinae represents the most important postural muscles in the body and it is vital that to maintain a healthy spine there is muscular balance with the abdominal muscles. Weak abdominal muscles are a major factor in giving spinal pain and conditions. A useful way of 'energy balancing' these two groups of muscles is given in Book Two. There is, of course, no substitution for exercising daily to maintain the muscles' elasticity and strength. This is more important than ever now we spend much of our days with poor posture, either slumped over a computer or by doing repetitive actions on a factory floor.

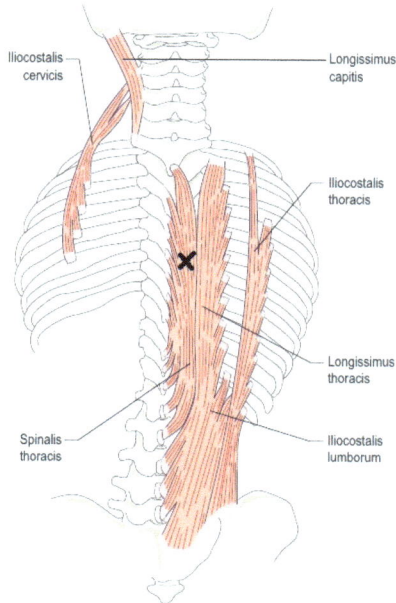

Figure 1.6.7 The Erector Spinae Muscle Group

Latissimus Dorsi (Figure 1.6.8)

This muscle will be discussed here, even though it affects the shoulder and lumbar spine, the muscle attachments are from the thoracic spine.

Origin – Insertion – Action It is a large, flat, triangular sheet of muscle extending from the sacral region to the upper arm. It originates by tendinous fibres of the spinous processes of T7-T12 anterior to the trapezius and from the lumbo-sacral fascia. It also has an origin in the lowest 4 ribs. The muscle inserts into the upper part of the humerus bone by a short tendon that has twisting fibres. It is a strong adductor, extensor and medial rotator of the arm. It also depresses the shoulder (with other muscles) and helps with

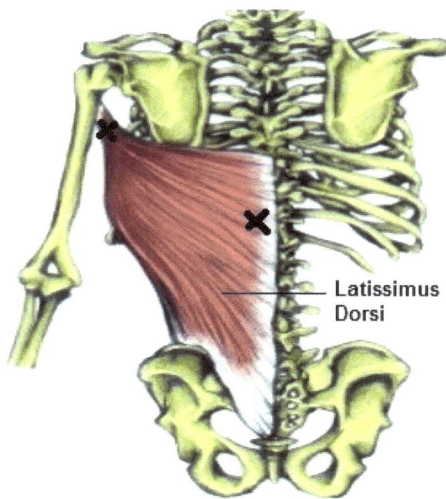

Figure 1.6.8 Latissimus Dorsi muscle

actions such as the down stroke in swimming. It also has a very important action in violent expiratory actions such as coughing and sneezing.

Nerve Supply It is innervated by the thoracodorsal nerve from C6, 7 and 8

Trigger Points This muscle may be affected by spasm and pain so can have numerous trigger points. The two that are highlighted are near its insertion at the arm and the mid thoracic region. The upper arm one may give pain down the arm, especially on the little finger side. The mid thoracic one acts like the erector spinae in giving symptoms, via the sympathetic nerves to the solar plexus region.

Holistic Considerations AK tells us that it is associated with Spleen energy – like its neighbour the Trapezius. In TCM the Spleen energy is linked with the pancreas. People with Type 1 diabetes may show a weakness in the Latissimus Dorsi giving a high shoulder on the weak side. The muscle also becomes weak when the patient has bad allergic reactions. One of the great thing about the muscle is its high nerve supply. If there is a mid to upper thoracic spinal trauma that affect the spinal cord, most of the muscles that are level or below the lesion become paralyzed. Due to its lower cervical innervation, this muscle will still act to assist the patient in wheelchair transfer and, in many case, to assist in walking retraining.

The Diaphragm (Figure 1.6.9)

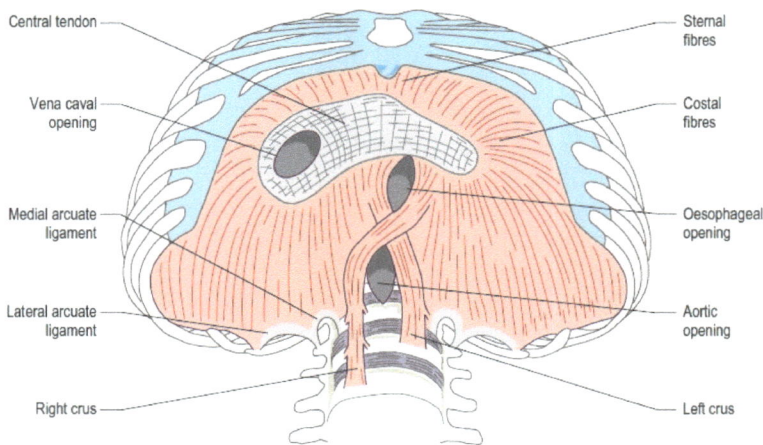

Figure 1.6.9 The Diaphragm Muscle

The diaphragm muscle is truly unique in that it is in the singular and is extremely important in so many ways. It is a broad muscle that separates the thoracic and abdominal cavities.

Origin – Insertion – Action Its muscular fibres attach to the back of the xiphoid process at the base of the sternum, its internal surfaces to the 7th-12th ribs. It is also attached to the Psoas Major muscle, L1 and L2 and the 12th rib. As you see from the diagram there are several openings to allow passage of the aorta, vena cava, oesophagus, splanchnic nerves and the sympathetic nerve trunks. It is, of course, the main muscle used in inspiration. It also has an important role in increasing intra-abdominal pressure working with the abdominal muscles in all expulsive act such as sneezing, coughing, laughing, shouting and singing as well as elimination of waste products.

Nerve Supply It is innervated with both motor and sensory nerves from the phrenic nerve (C3,4,5). Additional sensory fibres are from the lower six intercostal nerves.

Holistic Considerations In AK, the diaphragm is related to the Lung meridian (it couldn't be anything else) Due to its proximity with several important organs and vessels, it can be easily affected to produce pain and spasm. This may occur from irritation of the mid to lower thoracic spine that affects its sympathetic nerve supply. It may occur from respiratory or circulatory conditions or from stomach irritation due to excess acid. Diaphragmatic spasm is very painful and frightening. There are several more 'diaphragms' in the body – four in the central column and a total of eight altogether. These will be discussed in the next chapter. Also, discussed in Book Two will be several easy ways to ensure a relaxed diaphragm.

Lumbar and Sacral Muscles

There are several large and extremely important muscles at the lower end of the spine that help with stabilizing as well as flexing and side flexing, together with various actions on the lower limbs. The main muscles are the Iliopsoas group, Quadratus Lumborum, Gluteal group, Piriformis, and the muscles that make up the Abdominal group. I stress here that although the small vertebral interconnecting muscles such as the Multifidus, Rotatores, Interspinales and Intertransversarii haven't been described, they are, obviously very important and will be affected in virtually every treatment performed on the spine.

Iliopsoas Group – [Iliacus – Psoas Major – Psoas Minor] (Figure 1.6.10)

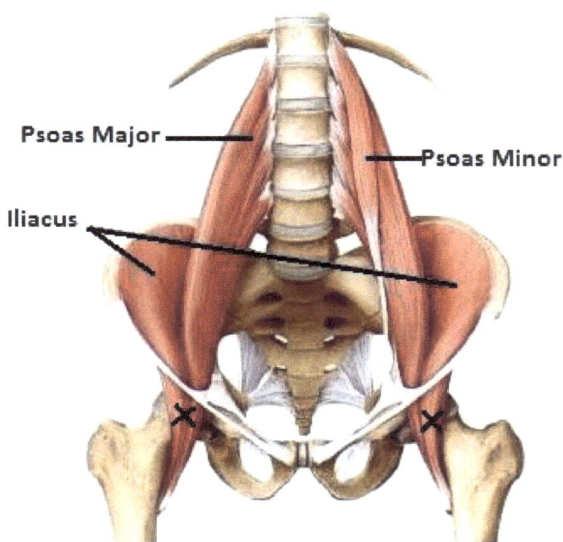

Figure 1.6.10 The Iliopsoas Group of Muscles

Origin – Insertion – Action The major muscles Psoas Major and Iliacus are usually grouped together as their insertion and actions are the same. The Psoas Minor tends to be a vestigial muscle and not present in everyone. The Psoas Major is large and strong and has its origin on the transverse processes of T12 and L1-5 as well as the sides of each of the bodies of the lumbar vertebrae, intermingling with the deep fascia surrounding the intervertebral discs. It descends through the inguinal ligament to insert on the lesser trochanter of the femur. The Iliacus has its origin on the anterior aspect of the pelvis and its fibres mingle with the Psoas Major near to its common insertion. The muscles flex and side flex the lumbar spine as well as flexing and medially rotating the femur.

Nerve Supply Both muscles are innervated from L1,2 and 3.

Trigger Points These muscles are very deep within the pelvic rim and although it is possible, with great pressure to feel the muscle as it passes through the pelvis, it is not advisable as there are many major blood vessels and nerves that may be bruised. The most important trigger point lies at the groin. Pain and spasm in this region may stem from other local muscles or irritation of the L1-2-3 discs. It may also come from the hip joint. Causes are sitting for long period (such as driving), suddenly rising from sitting or lying in the foetal position. Pain is felt the length of the lumbar spine up to the 12th rib and is a common type of back ache, often misconstrued as disc prolapse.

Holistic Considerations. In AK, the Iliopsoas is related to the energies of the Kidney, presumably as the kidney meridian lies very close. In my experience, though, they are more tied in with the Large Intestine meridian. Spasm of the iliacus may lead to abdominal pain centred around the appendix region and often gives rise to Ileo-caecal valve syndrome. Chronic and long-standing spasm of the Iliopsoas may give rise to the classic 'question mark' lumbar scoliosis. The treatment of this through touch therapy is described in Book Two.

Quadratus Lumborum (Figure 1.6.11)

Origin – Insertion – Action It is a large, flat, quadrilateral muscle and is relatively small but very important. It originates from the lower part of the 12th rib and from the transverse processes of L1,2,3 and 4. It inserts into the crest of the ilium. Its singular action is to side flex the spine and to stabilize the lower ribs, but when working together it extends the spine. It also stabilizes the lower rib cage and assists the diaphragm in breathing.

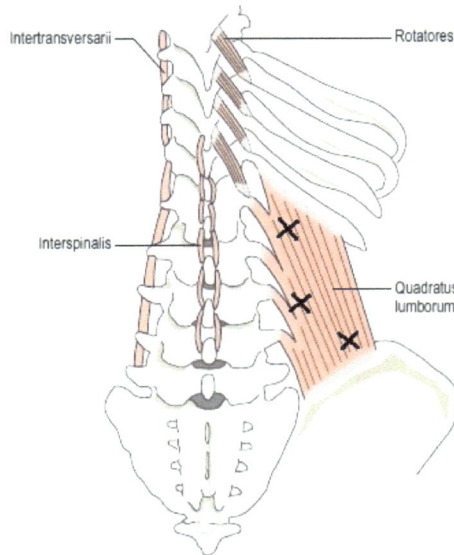

Figure 1.6.11 Quadratus Lumborum muscle

Nerve Supply It is innervated from T12, L1,2,3 and 4

Trigger Points This muscle is prone to spasm and pain due to its location. The causes could be trauma or chronic problems with the lumbar spine, respiratory imbalance, sacro-iliac or hip instability or bowel problems. There may be several trigger points on this muscle that give referred pain to the hips, pelvis and ape sciatic involvement. It is always essential to ease the spasm in this muscle in any low back syndromes. See Part Four to see how this is achieved.

Holistic Considerations This muscle is likely to become 'congested' with chronic bowel conditions. It is also affected with chronic hamstring problems (or vice versa). In AK, the associated organ/meridian is the large intestine.

Gluteal group [Gluteus Maximus, Gluteus Medius, Gluteal Minimus and Piriformis] (Figure 1.6.12)

Strictly speaking, only the Gluteus Maximus and Piriformis attach to the spine, at the sacrum. However, it is important to know these muscles as they do have an enormous influence on the spine and can give rise to a great deal of discomfort when in a state of imbalance.

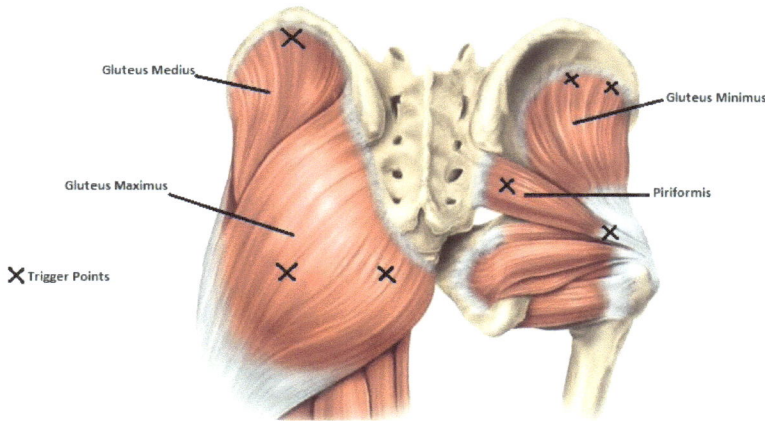

Figure 1.6.12 The Gluteal Muscles

Origin – Insertion – Action. The Gluteus maximus is attached to the postero-lateral aspect of the sacrum and coccyx and the posterior aspect of the iliac crest and inserts into the gluteal tuberosity of the femur as well as the iliotibial tract on the lateral aspect of the femur. The Gluteus Medius and Gluteus Minimus originate from the posterior aspect of the ilium and insert into the greater trochanter of the femur. The Piriformis originates from the lateral aspect of the sacrum and inserts into the greater trochanter. Although their individual actions vary, they generally extend, abduct and inwardly rotate the leg.

Nerve Supply This ranges from L4 to S3 depending on the muscle

Trigger Points As you can see from the diagram, several possible trigger points may exist on the gluteals. The Gluteus maximus is the most superficial of these muscles and its trigger points are very easy to note. To find the others requires more than a little pressure. When these knots appear in the muscles, pain and discomfort can vary enormously depending on the muscle and the individual. Pain is usually down the leg – often giving a sciatic referral. For the deeper muscles of the Medius, Minimus and Piriformis, pain is often very acute and felt around the lumbo-sacral junction and the hip. In fact, pain in the hip joint is a very common referral from Piriformis spasm. The cause is trauma and chronic conditions of the lower lumbar vertebrae as well as deviation of the coccyx.

Holistic Considerations Applied Kinesiology gives the 'Circulation-Sex' (CX) as the associated meridian. The correct word should be 'Pericardium' – I grew up with the term 'Heart Constrictor'. It is a member of the Fire Element and is associated with the Triple Energizer meridian. I realize why Kinesiologists reckon that the CX meridian is linked to the gluteal muscles, but I think it is a nonsense. Firstly, the term Circulation-Sex was coined by kinesiologists who did not change the words even though the world health authority standardised all the acupuncture nomenclature in 2005. Secondly, the practicalities are incorrect. These muscles should be linked to Bladder energy. Details of practical work in Book Two.

The Abdominals – [Rectus Abdominus – Obliquus Externus Abdominus -Obliquus Internus Abdominus – Transverse Abdominus] (Figure 1.6.13)

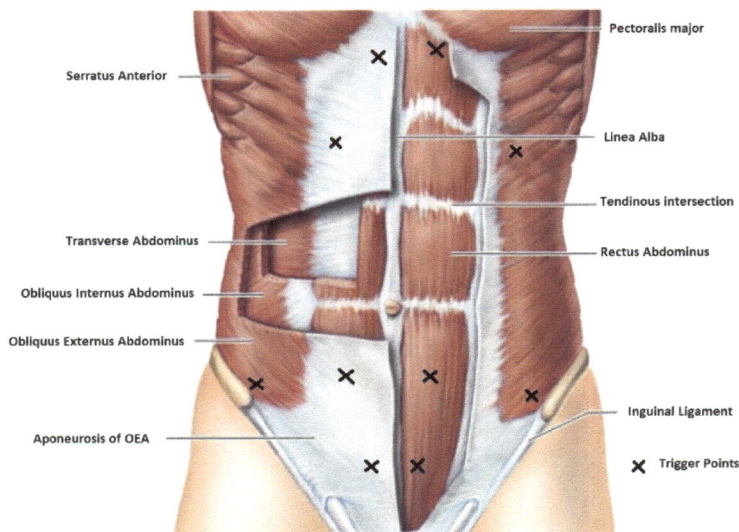

Figure 1.6.13 The Abdominal Group of Muscles

This final group of muscles that flex and rotate the trunk are probably the most important muscles in the body that have an influence over the wellbeing of the spine. This is despite none of them being attached to the spine. Weak abdominal muscles are amongst the most common reasons for weakness of the spine. There are several muscles that make up the frontal part of the torso, but we only need discuss four of them in detail, as they are the most important to us as therapists.

Rectus Abdominus

Origin – Insertion This is a long vertical muscle divided from each other by the central fascia known as the Linea Alba and intersected by 3 horizontal fibrous bands known as Tendinous Intersections. This muscle is colloquially known as the '6-pack'. It originates at the superior aspect of the symphysis pubis and inserts on the 5th, 6th and 7th costal cartilages and by fascia to the inferior aspect of the sternum at the xiphoid.

Nerve Supply – Innervated by T6-T12 (ventral rami)

Trigger Points – There are 3 areas on this muscle that are prone to trigger points, due to weakness in the spinal region, constipation, exercising too vigorously, excessive coughing or scar tissue post-surgery. The upper trigger points give pain referral to the stomach region (internally) giving bloating and heartburn plus spinal discomfort: the middle trigger points often give referral to the lower abdomen and uterus and are especially important in relieving menstrual discomfort (period pain): the middle right trigger point sometimes gives pain to the appendix region: the lower trigger points will give referred pain to the lower lumbar, sacrum and sacro-iliac region.

Transverse Abdominus

Origin – Insertion This is the innermost muscle and has horizontal fibres. It is attached laterally to the lateral third of the inguinal ligament, the iliac crest, the thoracolumbar fascia, the 12th rib and intermingles with the diaphragm. It inserts into the linea alba, public crest and intermingles with the Obliquus Internus muscle.

Nerve Supply This muscle is innervated from the ventral rami of T7 to T12 and L1

Trigger Points This muscle is too deep for any trigger points it may have to be treated manually but the symptoms they give are the same as the Obliquus muscles.

Obliquus Externus Abdominus

Origin – Insertion It is the most superficial of all the abdominals and is the strongest of the 3 diagonal muscles. It originates from the lower eight ribs and their costal cartilages, and from the sternum via an aponeurosis (fascial sheet). It inserts into the inguinal ligament via a large aponeurosis (see diagram) that extends from the pelvic crest to the symphysis ligament.

Nerve Supply Ventral rami of T7-T12

Trigger Points These can be many and various. Two regions are prominent is having trigger points – just by the lower rib insertion and in the groin by the iliac crest. The causes were described with the previous muscle. The symptoms are heartburn and pseudo hiatus hernia type discomfort (GORD) with the upper one and pain in the groin, testicles and inner leg with the lower one.

Obliquus Internus Abdominus

Origin – Insertion This muscle lies deep to the Externus muscle. Distally and laterally it is attached to the inguinal ligament, iliac crest and thoraco-lumbar fascia. It inserts by blending in with the Transverse Abdominus and with the lower three ribs.

Nerve Supply Ventral rami of T6-T12

Trigger Points They exist and give similar symptoms to the other in this muscle group but lie deep so difficulty in treating them mechanically.

Actions of the Abdominal Group They have three main actions, to flex and rotate the trunk, to help in explosive actions such as vomiting, coughing, sneezing, defecation, childbirth etc. and to assist in respiration with the diaphragm. Anyone who has had abdominal surgery will appreciate how weak these muscles become in a very short time and how difficult the explosive actions are. As stated before it is essential that these muscles are kept as strong as possible (within constraints of age etc.) to keep the spine as strong and mobile as possible.

Holistic Considerations of the Group Applied Kinesiology tells us that this group is related to Small Intestine energy. This makes a lot of sense as weakness in these muscles can give rise to abdominal symptoms such as bloating, GORD, ileo-caecal valve syndrome, constipation and abdominal discomfort. This is obviously a two-way event with any of these conditions, if not treated, can give rise to muscle congestion and weakness. The Rectus Abdominus may become affected during pregnancy when the linea alba stretches to allow foetal growth. Following childbirth, this fascial ligament doesn't always heal and can give rise to 'large stomach syndrome' as if the woman is once again pregnant. The same may occur in abdominal surgery. The condition is call 'diastasis recti'. There are several ways to help this condition but it is essential that the 'core' stability of the lower body is maintained and strengthened by exercise modules such as Pilates. As stated before, the abdominals are the antagonists of the erector spinae – when one group is weak, the other is affected, so it is important also to strengthen the erector spinae as well.

Chapter Seven – The Major Spinal Chakras

The chakra energy system has been a study of mine for more years than I care to remember, and I maintain that it is the most comprehensive and far reaching of all the subtle energy philosophies. The system is complicated, but once learnt and absorbed, it will become your friend and ally, even when tackling chronic and complicated conditions. This chapter will, of course, concentrate on the spinal chakras but in the practical section in Book Two, some of the frontal major chakras as well as the minor chakras will be utilised. The word *chakra* is Sanskrit for *wheel*. They are said to be *force centres* or *whorls of energy* permeating from a point on the physical body through the various layers of the subtle body of our aura in an ever-increasing fan shaped formation. Although a study of the chakras isn't complete without studying the complete aura, for the purposes of this book, all that is required is knowledge of the lower energy matrix that consists of the Physical, Etheric and Emotional Bodies.

The Aura (Figure 1.7.1)

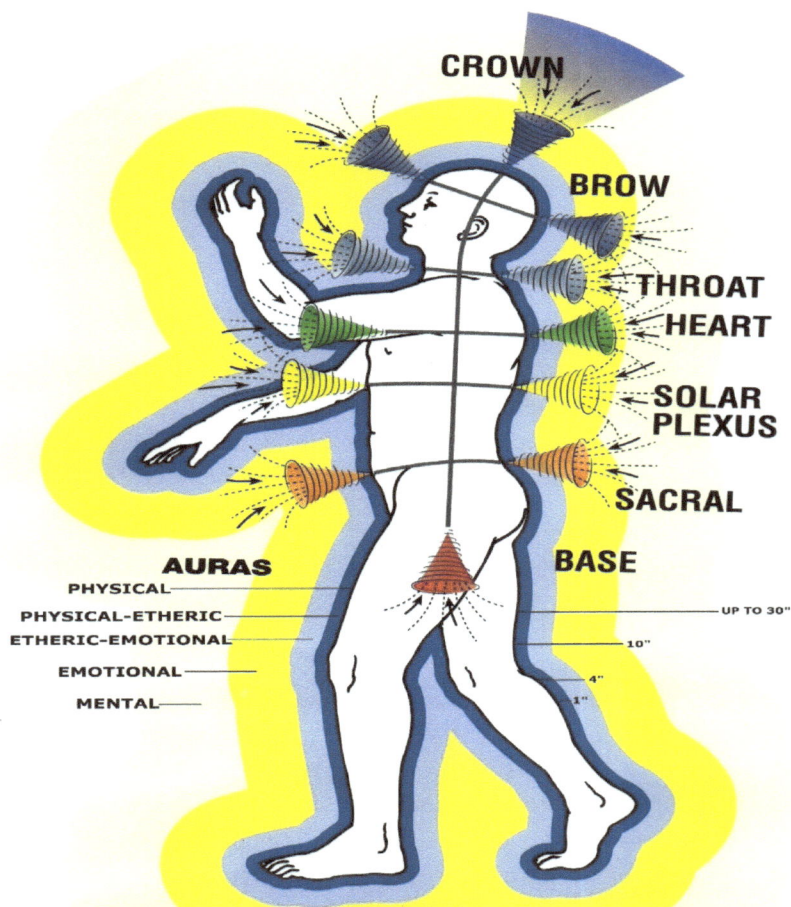

Figure 1.7.1 The Aura and Major Chakras

There are said to be seven bodies, including the Physical Body, that make up our aura. They are Physical, Etheric, Emotional or Astral, Mental, Intuitional, Monadic and Divine or Spiritual. Different philosophies, individuals and cultures have given these bodies other names depending on whether they are discussed as part of Eastern religion, Hindu, Buddhist, Western Spiritual or New Age terms. Some very gifted people have the capability of seeing and interpreting auras (clairvoyants), some can feel them but not see them and other just see different colours. Many children up to the age of seven see some type of aura. The acceptance of the auras are fundamental precepts in being able to learn about the chakras, not only when used with yoga and meditation, but also when performing subtle bodywork. Chakras simply do not make sense without incorporating them into the study of the aura.

Physical Body

Looking at the body from a purely esoteric viewpoint, it can truthfully be said that all the Physical Body does is to house our symptoms. A Yogi or even a classically trained homoeopath would not be interested in the Physical Body – all they need to know are our emotions and personalities. I firmly believe that most of our chronic ills are tied up with the emotions and the symptoms of dis-ease are merely housed in the Physical Body in order that we, as practitioners, can make a discernible assessment and diagnosis of the true cause (aetiology) of the condition. Once that is known, it is the *cause* that is treated. When we utilise the chakra system (often combined with other systems) we can be assured that it is the cause of the condition that has been addressed.

Etheric Body

The word *etheric* comes from *ether*, meaning the state between energy and matter. This first 'invisible' body can be seen by most people given the correct training in tuning in to the vibrations that it exudes. Strictly, there are two parts to it, the Physical-Etheric and the Etheric-Emotional. The outer limit of these are approximately 1" (25mm) and 4 "(100mm). This body consists of a network of fine tubular threadlike channels known as the nadis. These seem to be related to the cerebrospinal fluid, endocrine system and the autonomic nervous system. This Body is a receiver, assimilator and transmitter of vital force via the chakras.

Emotional Body

The third body is called the Emotional or Astral Body due to its involvement with our emotions. Its outer border follows roughly the shape of the Etheric Body with an outer border of between 10" - 12" (250 – 300mm). Multitudes of different changes are constantly taking place within this subtle body, though we are usually unaware of these. Each of us is bombarded by stimuli from both external and internal sources. The main function of this body is to act like a filtration system of thoughts (from the Mental Body) and negative processes from the Etheric – via the major chakras. Imbalance within this body will eventually give us symptoms on the physical.

For a full description of the aura, please see my *book 'Healing with the Chakra Energy System – Acupressure, Bodywork and Reflexology for Total Health'* – North Atlantic Books- Berkeley, USA (2006)

The Chakras

It is thought that the discovery of chakras stems from Ayurvedic medical philosophy developed over five thousand years ago, it therefore seems to be more established that Traditional Chinese Medicine. As with TCM, though, the study of the chakras is a lifelong pursuit. No one person can ever hope to have a monopoly on the total ramifications of the chakra energy system. Due to their esoteric and complex nature, much mysticism surrounds them and what I have attempted to do over the past thirty-five years is to make them more accessible and easily understood by the practitioner. Each of the seven major chakras is different in form, make up, colour and vibration. There are said to be seven major chakras, twenty-one minor chakras and over seven hundred micro chakras that we know as acupuncture points. Some authorities state that there are many more than seven major chakras, some giving as many as twelve.

Some of these are considered to be wholly 'off-body' and do not create the 'link' between the physical 'us' and our emotions, mental and spiritual make up as the seven majors chakras do. Some authorities place them only on the front of the body and some just on the spine. I have always considered them to have both anterior and posterior aspect. Indeed, I consider that our auric energy girdles the physical body with concentrations at the various horizontal 'diaphragms'. The anterior and posterior major chakras are focal points on these diaphragmatic regions. Figure 1.7.2 shows the lower six major spinal chakras showing their spinal influences (colour co-ordinated) and their diaphragm regions. The anterior major chakras generally deal with more chronic illness, whilst the spinal ones deal with acute and musculo-skeletal imbalance. This is purely because the anterior energy channels are 'yin' in nature and the posterior ones are 'yang'. In practice, though, one can easily treat both acute and chronic imbalance from either anterior or spinal chakras.

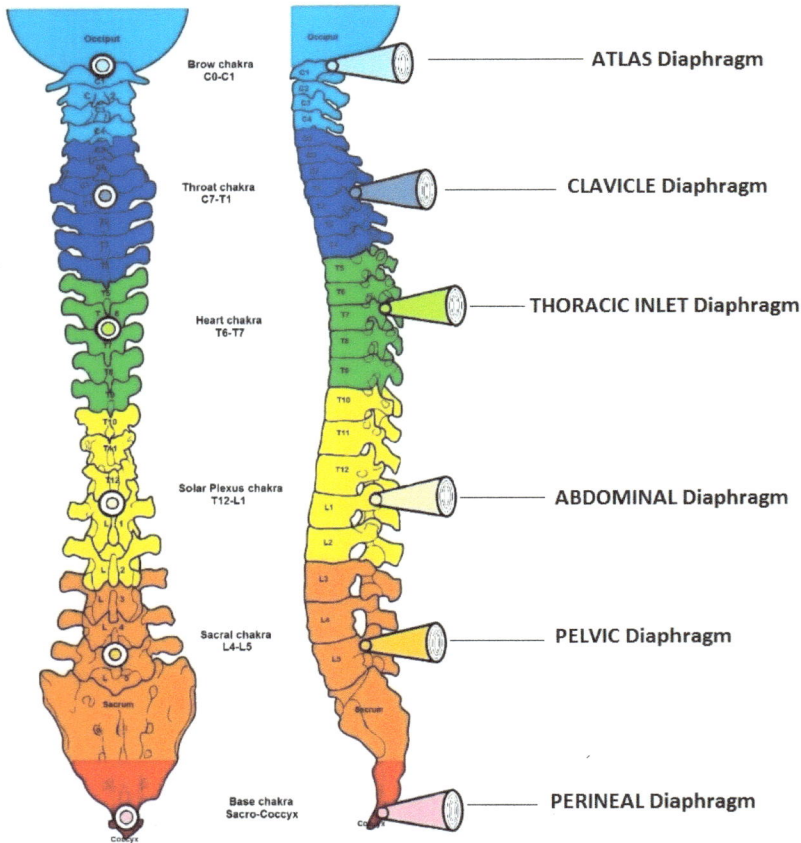

Figure 1.7.2 The Seven Major Chakras and their Spinal Influence – showing the 'diaphragms'

Esoteric Formation of the Spinal Chakras

Although TCM and Ayurvedic medicine originate from different ages and roots, it is possible to combine the two philosophies so as explain the origin of chakras. In Ayurvedic medicine the etheric aura is filled with thousands of energy channels called *nadis* through which the vital force (prana) flows. Through this extensive network of subtle channels the chakras are connected to the physical body. Congestion of the nadis with stagnant energy (from within or without) affects the physical body which then gives us physical symptoms. The nadis are interwoven with the nervous system, and because of this, they affect the nature and quality of nerve transmission within the brain, spinal cord and peripheral nerves. The three main nadis components that are aligned on the vertical axis of the body (anterior and posterior) are the *Sushumna, Ida* and *Pingala*. Most traditional texts agree that the Sushumna nadi is only situated along the spinal cord and is the main channel for the flow of nervous energy up and down the spine. From the Sushumna nadi, thousands of minor nadis branch out and link with the nervous system in the physical body. We can therefore equate the Sushumna as the equivalent of the Governor (Du Mai) meridian. The Ida nadi is aligned on the left side parallel with the central line and the Pingala is situated on the right. A chakra is formed when twenty-one nadis intersect. I have equated the posterior aspects of the Ida and Pingala nadi with the Inner Bladder Line meridians. Traditional Indian and Tibetan medicine have the coiled serpent (caduceus) weaving its way through the three main nadis, and a chakra is formed where the coils intersect. The 'crossing over' aspect resembles the modern medical emblem or logo of the medical and healing professions (I have it on my logo). Ida is associated with coolness, the right-brain hemisphere and the parasympathetic nervous system, whereas Pingala is associated with heat, the left-brain hemisphere and the sympathetic nervous system. The crossover occurs at the main horizontal 'diaphragmatic' regions (see previous section). It is also at these regions that there are connections with the endocrine glands and autonomic nervous system, that, in my humble opinion are energised via the etheric body. I also maintain that the Sushumna nadis energy equates to cerebrospinal fluid flow. In my experience, whether the links are energetic, reflected, trigger or nervous does not matter! I have spent three decades trying to figure this one out – it is what it is! Figure 1.7.3 shows a diagrammatic representation of the TCM approach with the Governor and Bladder meridian with the acupoints; Figure 1.7.4 the Ayurvedic approach with the Sushumna, Ida and Pingala nadis with the named chakras; Figure 1.7.5 the Caduceus energies of intertwining; Figure 1.7.6 shows an emblem of the caduceus combined with the Chinese Monad of Yin/Yang and Figure 1.7.7 shows my own logo.

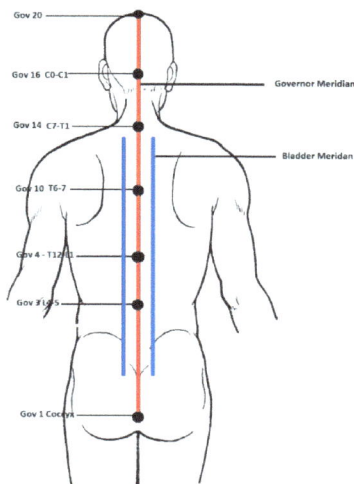

Figure 1.7.3 TCM meridians and acupoints

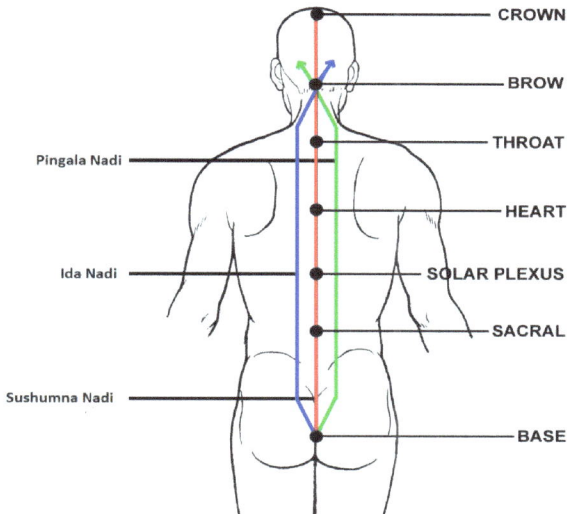

Figure 1.7.4 Ayurvedic Nadis and Chakras

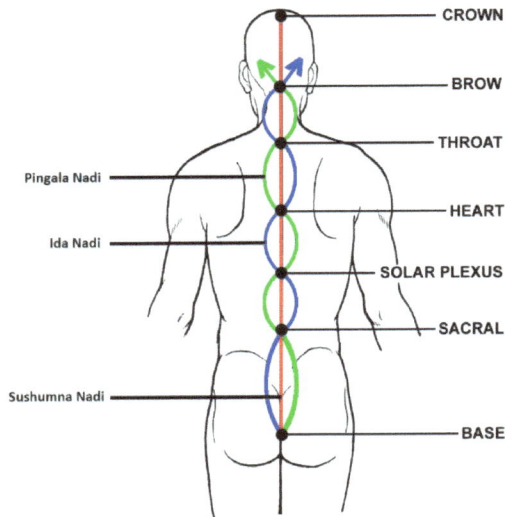

Figure 1.7.5 The Nadis in the Caduceus Formation with the Spinal Chakras

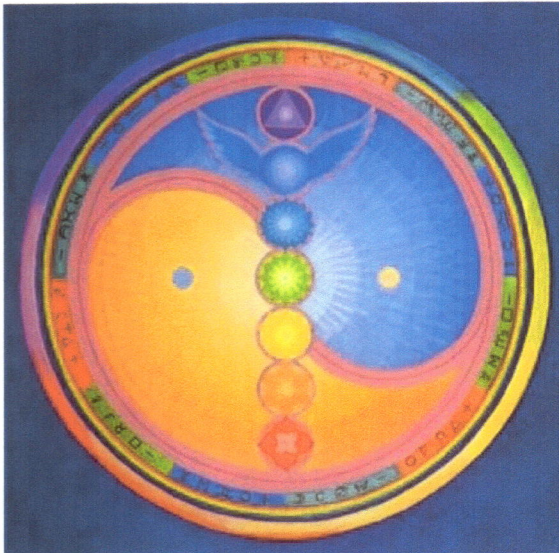

Figure 1.7.6 A typical Symbol of the Caduceus and the Yin/Yang symbol of TCM

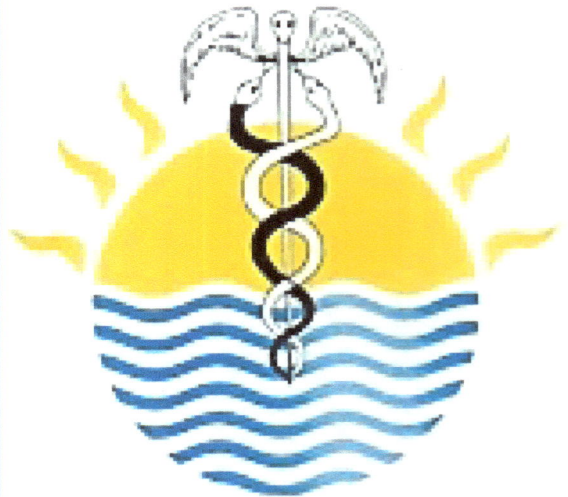

Figure 1.7.7 My Personal Logo

Structure

The structure of each of the chakras is different from Crown through to Base and differs with age of the individual. Its general shape can be likened to an inverted ice cream cone (see Figure 1.7.8), with the narrow end 'attached' to the physical body via the 'pea soup' conglomeration of nadis at the physical-etheric level. The size of a chakra at the outer border of the Etheric Body is approximately two inches (5 cms); at the outer border of the Emotional Body is the size of an average saucer; and at the outer border of the Mental Body it is the size of a dinner plate. There is, therefore, much intermingling of energy with two adjacent chakras. The Crown and Base chakras in a baby are shaped like those of an adult, whereas the middle five are small and round as they do not fully function until the child reaches the age of seven or thereabouts.

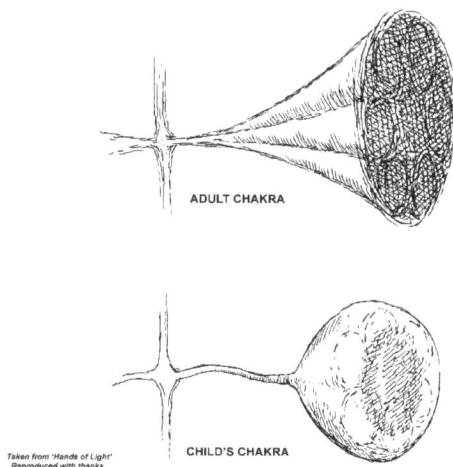

ADULT CHAKRA

Taken from 'Hands of Light'
Reproduced with thanks

CHILD'S CHAKRA

Figure 1.7.8 Diagrammatic interpretation of the shape of a typical chakra

The Base (or Root or Muladhara) chakra is said to deal with conceptual and ancestral energy, and at the top end, the Crown (or Sahasrara) deals with our spirituality. At the age of seven the Sacral chakra is fully functional, followed by the Solar Plexus and so on, at the age of approximately fifteen, all the major chakras have assumed the iconic cone shape. In the body of each chakra are four or more components of rotating, cylindrically shaped vortices. It is these individual components that vibrate and resonate to a certain frequency and vibration that is unique to each individual chakra. The lower chakras resonate somewhat slowly, whilst the Brow and Crown resonate very quickly.

Chakra Functions and States of Imbalance

There is much debate on what the chakras do, but the consensus is that they have three main functions: -

- To vitalise and harmonise the Physical, Etheric and Emotional bodies
- To facilitate the development of self-consciousness
- To transmit spiritual energy, thereby bringing the individual into a state of spiritual being.

The first two may be undertaken by a person using yoga, meditation, martial art or self-healing, or by a practitioner/therapist using the same approaches plus acupuncture, acupressure, reflexology, colour, sound to name but a few. The third function remains the purview of the meditation arts or yoga.

There are three states of imbalance – Congestion, Over-stimulation and Incoordination

Congestion occurs when energy is not allowed to flow freely. This occurs when there is sluggishness of vital force in a region that in turn affects the lymphatic drainage, blood flow, nerve stimulation or flow of CSF. The process may occur from within outwards or outward to within. Examples would be consuming too much saturated fat that, in turn, causes congestion in the stomach and small intestine and eventually the skin, lymph flow and endocrine irregularity. This would affect the Solar Plexus and Throat chakras. Another example would be where invading microorganisms give rise to congestion in the Throat chakra, causing lymphatic congestion in the tonsils and other parts of the immune system.

Overstimulation A chakra can become overstimulated when too much energy is drawn into and through it. A fever is an example of an overactive point of energy that is trying to disperse and flow outward into physical expression. An over enthusiastic libido causes overstimulation in the Base and Sacral chakras. Someone working constantly under fluorescent lighting will have an overstimulated Brow chakra, resulting in headaches and dizziness.

Incoordination This occurs between two associated chakras, creating a weakness in one of them, that eventually results in poor health. If the physical and etheric counterparts of a chakra aren't well integrated, then debilitation and devitalisation will occur. When a chakra becomes congested or overstimulated, it seeks support from its coupled chakra, which, in turn, may cause symptoms there. An example would be where impotence causes an imbalance between the Sacral and Throat chakras.

Associations and Correspondences Each of the major chakras has many associations and correspondences. They are the: -

- Vertebral level and its acupoint
- Spinal influence
- Coupled major chakra
- Coupled minor chakra
- Endocrine gland
- Internal organ
- Key points
- Meridians
- Muscles
- Autonomic nerves
- Emotional/mental
- Spiritual
- Colour and Sound

In addition to the above, described below, there are associations to Element; Gemstone; Essential oil; Crystal; Earth energy; Planet and Metal. I am positive that there are more than these but are quite obscure.

Vertebral Level, Acupoint and Spinal Influence

Base (Muladhara) chakra is situated at Gov 1, at the tip of the coccyx. However, this acupoint is not used for obvious anatomical reasons. As there is an area of influence in acupressure, acupoint Gov 2 is used for the spinal Base chakra. This is situated at the sacro-coccyx junction and is much more 'acceptable' than Gov 1. It is, however, essential that the patient is warned each time you place your fingers in that region. The Base chakra influences the coccyx and the lower half of the sacrum.

Sacral (Svadhistana) chakra is situated at the junction of L4-5 between the spinous processes. The acupuncture point is Gov 3. The spinal influence is L3, L4, L5 and the upper part of the sacrum.

Solar Plexus (Manipura) chakra is situated at the junction of T12 and L1 between their spinous processes. The acupuncture point is Gov 6 and the spinal influence is T10, T11, T12, L1 and L2.

Heart (Anahata) chakra is situated at the centre of the thoracic spine between the spinous processes of T6-T7. The acupuncture point is Gov 10 and its spinal influence is T5, T6, T7, T8 and T9.

Throat (Vishuddha) chakra is situated between the spinous processes of C7 – T1. The acupuncture point is Gov 14 and its spinal influence is C5, C6, C7, T1, T2, T3 and T4.

<u>Brow</u> (Ajna) chakra is situated between the base of the occiput and the atlas bone C0 – C1. The acupuncture point is Gov 16 and its spinal influence is the Occiput, C1, C2, C3 and C4.

<u>Crown</u> (Sahasrara) chakra is not situated on the spine but at the top of the head at Gov 20. The skull influences are the frontal, parietal, ethmoid and sphenoid bones.

Coupled Major and Minor Chakras

These are important relationships in practical therapy, especially when performing acupressure and reflexology. They are clinically important as well – when a chakra is congested or over active, its associated chakra comes to the rescue in helping. This, of course, is a two-edged sword, as symptoms of the associated chakra will often ensue. The minor chakras and their location have been one of my many research projects into this esoteric form of healing. They are 'minor' because they are not as powerful or influential as the seven major chakras, but, in turn, they are more powerful and have more influence than 'ordinary' acupoints. There are 21 minor chakras, although the Spleen chakra is recognised in some quarters as being the eighth major. Then other twenty minor chakras are bilateral i.e. ten on each side of the body. Figure 1.7.9 shows the anterior and posterior major chakras as well as the minor chakras and their locations. The couples are as follows: -

Major Chakra	Coupled Major Chakra	Coupled Minor Chakra	Coupled Minor Chakra
CROWN	BASE	FOOT	HAND
BROW	BASE	CLAVICULAR	GROIN
THROAT	SACRAL	SHOULDER	NAVEL
HEART	SOLAR PLEXUS	EAR	INTERCOSTAL
SOLAR PLEXUS	HEART	SPLEEN	-
SACRAL	THROAT	SPLEEN	-
BASE	CROWN	ELBOW	KNEE

Please note that the Base chakra is the couple of both the Crown and Brow and that the Solar Plexus and Sacral have just the one couple – Spleen chakra. The Spleen chakra is the only non-peripheral minor chakra and is sometimes referred to as the eighth major. The subject of the Minor Chakras has not been explained fully in any book I have read. I intend to put that right in a future tome – watch this space!

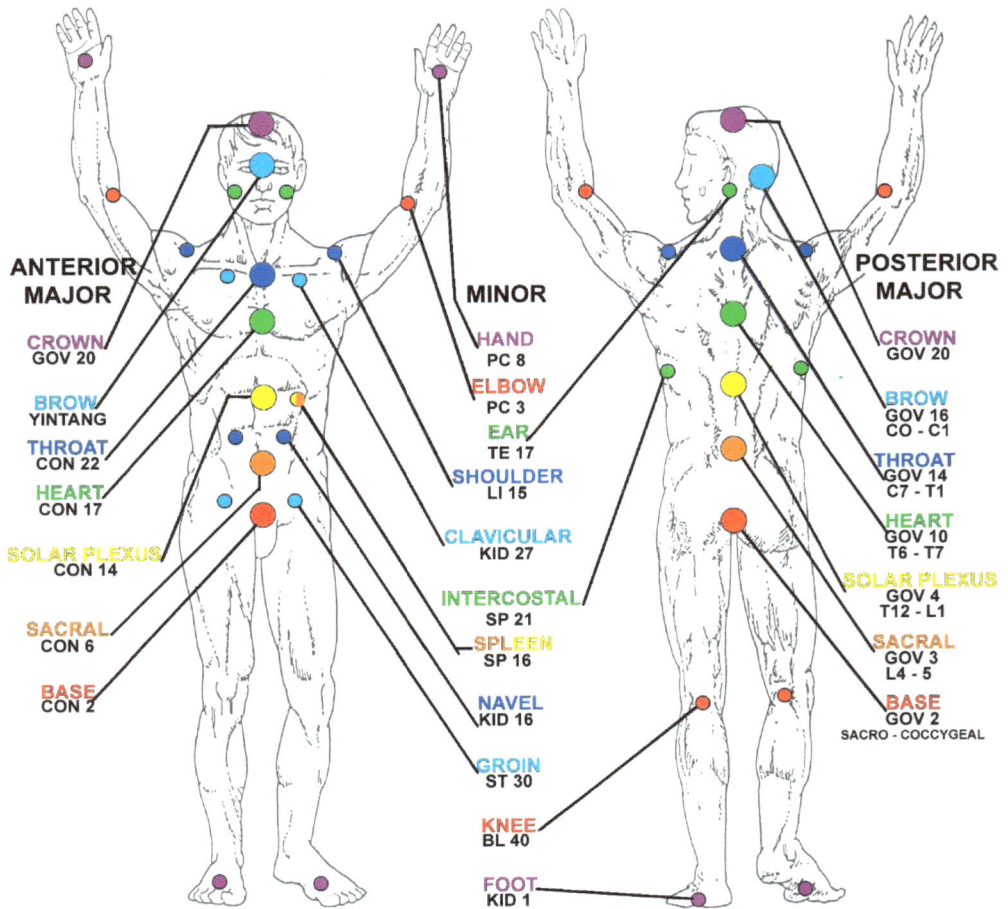

Figure 1.7.9 The Major and Minor Chakras and their Couples – Colour Coordinated

Associated Endocrine Glands

This relationship is extremely important in both clinical knowledge and practical application. Although this couple is dealt with rather scantily in the more esoteric publications, it is one of the most concrete associations that can be reproduced on a practical level again and again to give spectacular clinical results. The endocrine glands are parts of the physical body and have nerve, blood, lymph and energy links with the rest of the physical body and yet produce chemicals (hormones) that are extremely powerful in affecting all the auric bodies as well as the physical. The links are as follows: -

- The CROWN chakra is associated with the PINEAL gland
- The BROW chakra is associated with the PITUITARY gland
- The THROAT chakra is associated with the THYROID and PARATHYROID glands
- The HEART chakra is associated with the THYMUS gland
- The SOLAR PLEXUS chakra is associated with the PANCREAS gland
- The SACRAL chakra is associated with the OVARIES and TESTES
- The BASE chakra is associated with the ADRENAL MEDULLA and ADRENAL CORTEX

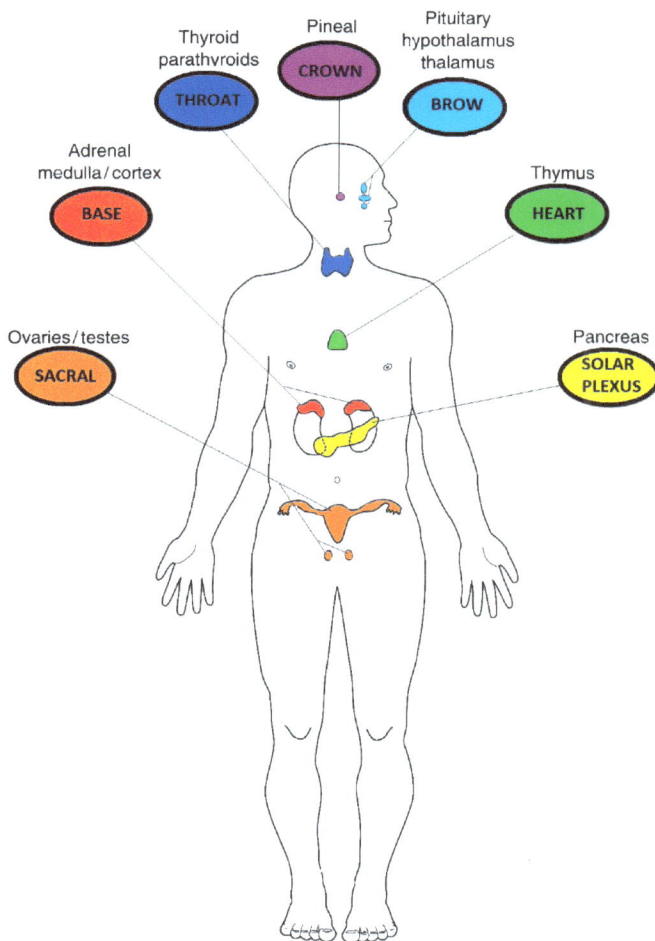

Figure 1.7.10 The Spinal Chakras and Endocrine Glands

Since these links first appeared in my book 'Healing with the Chakra Energy System' (NAB – 2006), I have received many comments about their locations. Let me assure these folk that the Crown chakra *is* associated with the Pineal and *not* the Pituitary – and vice versa. I also appreciate that the Base chakra appears to be out of phase with the Sacral regarding its anatomical positioning. Once again, let me reassure those who disagree with me that I have used these links for over thirty years in treating patients – and *they are correct*. The adrenal glands happen to be anatomically superior to the uterus and pancreas – that's an anatomical fact but it makes no difference to its associated chakra. (Figure 1.7.10 refers)

Associated Internal Organ

Each of the major chakras is associated with one or more internal organ or parts of the body. This link is probably via the autonomic nervous system.

- The CROWN chakra is associated with the upper brain (higher functions) and the right eye.
- The BROW chakra is associated with the lower brain (central nervous system), ears, nose and left eye.

- The THROAT chakra is associated with the lungs, bronchus, throat, larynx, pharynx, upper part of the lymphatic system and the large intestine.
- The HEART chakra is associated with the heart, blood circulation, middle lymphatics and the vagus (parasympathetic) nerve
- The SOLAR PLEXUS chakra is associated with the stomach, liver, gall bladder, spleen, pancreas and the duodenal/jejunum parts of the small intestine
- The SACRAL chakra is associated with the reproductive system, lower lymphatics and the ileum part of the small intestine
- The BASE chakra is associated with the spinal column, kidneys, bladder, urethra and ureters.

The Key Points

For those of you who are versed in traditional acupuncture, you will know that each of the eight extraordinary meridians has its Key point. This is a point, situated on the limbs that 'opens up' the meridian to use it. My early research into the chakra energy system in the mid 1970's found that each of the major and minor chakras has its own Key points that work in a similar way. When using the chakra energy system with acupuncture, it is essential to needle the Key point first. Each major chakra has two Key points (one on the periphery and one on the Governor or Conception meridians) and each minor chakra has just one. When this system is used with acupressure and reflexology (as in this book), they balance the chakra and become a part of the treatment. Also, when using touch therapy, it is essential to use the peripheral Key point, whilst the spinal/central Key point may be use as a 'backup'. The backup points are given in brackets. There are some instances though, when using the major chakra to treat spinal conditions that the Key points may be superfluous. These will be outlined in Book Two. Diagrams showing the location of the Key points will be given in the descriptions of each specific chakra. The Key points are as follows: -

- The CROWN chakra Key point is TE 5 (Con 4)
- The BROW chakra Key point is SP 6 (Gov 4)
- The THROAT chakra Key point is LR 5 (Con 6)
- The HEART chakra Key point is HT 1 (Gov 7)
- The SOLAR PLEXUS chakra Key point is TE 4 (Con 17)
- The SACRAL chakra Key point is PC 3 (Gov 12)
- The BASE chakra Key point is LR 8 (Con 22)

Associated Meridians

Each of the major chakras is related to one, two or three meridians. The meridians may be used as supplementary treatment or at the commencement of a treatment session by stroking the meridian in the direction of energy flow. The links (that will be shown graphically when the individual chakra is described) are as follows: -

- The CROWN chakra is associated with the TRIPLE ENERGIZER meridian
- The BROW chakra is associated with the GALL BLADDER meridian
- The THROAT chakra is associated with the LUNG and LARGE INTESTINE meridians
- The HEART chakra is associated with the HEART and SMALL INTESTINE meridians
- The SOLAR PLEXUS chakra is associated with the LIVER and STOMACH meridians
- The SACRAL chakra is associated with the SPLEEN and PERICARDIUM meridians
- The BASE chakra is associated with the BLADDER and KIDNEY meridians

There are also associations to the eight extraordinary meridians, but these are generally the reserve of the anterior major chakras.

Associated muscles

The treatment of musculo-skeletal condition is just one aspect of this amazing system of medicine, and is the one that most 'hands – on' practitioners use. As has been detailed earlier in Part Two, Applied Kinesiology and Touch For Health has given us the integration of muscles and meridians as well as organic-muscle relationships. My own pioneering work has taken this one stage further by relating each muscle with the major and minor chakras. In practical terms, muscles may now be strengthened, weakened or simply treated in a very rapid way by balancing the muscle with its related chakra. Below is a list of associated muscles, organ, meridian, vertebra, major chakra and minor chakra. You will notice that each muscle has a different combination, and that the Throat and Sacral chakras are extremely important in this work. Details of how to use this information in a practical way will be given in Part Four where this table will be replicated.

Muscle	Organ/Body	Meridian	Vertebra	Major Chakra	Minor Chakra
Sternomastoid	Sinus	Stomach	C1	Crown	Ear
Facial Muscles	Sinus	Governor	C1-2	Crown	Ear
Neck, ant. post.	Sinus	Stomach	C1,2,3	Brow	Clavicular
Upper Trapezius	Eye and Ear	Kidney	C3	Crown	Ear
Supraspinatus	Brain	Conception	C4	Crown	Ear
Levator Scapula	Parathyroid gland	Stomach	C5	Throat	Clavicular
Pectoralis Maj. (clavicular)	Stomach	Stomach	C6	Throat	Shoulder
Pectoralis Maj. (Sternal)	Liver	Liver	C6	Throat	Clavicular
Biceps	Stomach	Stomach	C6	Throat	Elbow
Serratus Anterior	Lung	Lung	C6	Throat	Shoulder
Subscapularis	Heart	Heart	C6	Throat	Shoulder
Infraspinatus	Thymus gland	Triple Energiser	C6	Throat	Shoulder
Brachialis	Stomach	Stomach	C6	Throat	Elbow
Brachioradialis	Stomach	Stomach	C6	Throat	Hand
Wrist Extensors	Stomach	Stomach	C6	Throat	Hand
Triceps	Pancreas	Spleen	C7	Throat	Elbow
Middle and Lower Trapezius	Spleen	Spleen	C7	Throat	Shoulder
Supinator	Stomach	Stomach	C7	Throat	Hand
Latissimus Dorsi	Pancreas	Spleen	C7	Throat	Intercostal
Wrist Flexors	Stomach	Stomach	C7	Throat	Hand
Deltoid	Lung	Lung	T1	Throat	Shoulder
Teres Major	Spine	Governor	T1	Throat	Elbow
Teres Minor	Thyroid	Triple Energiser	T1	Throat	Elbow
Rhomboids	Liver	Liver	T2-L3	Throat	Hand
Sacrospinalis	Bladder	Bladder	T4-T12	Heart	Intercostal
Abdominals	Small Intestine	Small Intestine	L1-2	Solar Plexus	Navel

Quadriceps	Small Intestine	Small Intestine	L2	Solar Plexus	Groin
Iliopsoas	Kidney	Kidney	L2	Sacral	Groin
Sartorius	Adrenals	Triple Energiser	L3	Sacral	Knee
Gracilis	Adrenals	Triple Energiser	L3	Sacral	Foot
Tibialis Anterior	Bladder	Bladder	L4	Sacral	Foot
Adductors	Circulation	Pericardium	L4-5	Sacral	Knee
Tensor Fascia Latae	Large Intestine	Large Intestine	L5	Sacral	Knee
Gluteus Medius	Sexual	Pericardium	L5	Sacral	Groin
Gluteus Maximus	Sexual	Pericardium	S1	Sacral	Knee
Hamstrings	Large Intestine	Large Intestine	S1	Sacral	Knee
Tibialis Posterior	Adrenals	Bladder	S1	Sacral	Foot
Peroneus Longus	Bladder	Bladder	S1	Sacral	Foot
Gastrocnemius/Soleus	Adrenals	Triple Energiser	S2	Sacral	Foot
Popliteus	Gall Bladder	Gall Bladder	S3	Sacral	Knee

Associated Autonomic Nerves

The association between the autonomic nervous system (ANS) and the chakras is of huge significance in practical complementary medicine. Most health care professionals agree that the ANS's role in maintaining good health is fundamental. I have discovered a link between the chakras and the individual nerve plexuses of the ANS. The links are as follows: -

- The CROWN chakra is not linked with the ANS
- The BROW chakra is linked with the Superior Cervical Ganglion
- The THROAT chakra is linked with the Inferior Cervical Ganglion
- The HEART chakra is linked with the Coeliac Plexus and Ganglion
- The SOLAR PLEXUS chakra is also linked with the Coeliac Plexus and Ganglion
- The SACRAL chakra is linked with the Inferior Mesenteric Ganglion
- The BASE chakra is linked with the Pelvic Plexus

Figure 1.7.11 shows this diagrammatically. I was tempted to place the spinal chakras superimposed onto a previous illustration but it would have made it too 'busy'. As usual, the practicalities of using this information with acupressure and reflexology is discussed in Book Two.

Associated Emotions and Spiritual

As has been stated many times, it is without doubt that our emotions are responsible for health changes and the chakra energy system may be used both in analysis and treatment with individual chakras. When patients exhibit certain emotional/mental traits it would indicate imbalance with the chakra and when that chakra is energy balanced and treated, the emotions are affected to enhance positivity within the system. Emotions are not 'black and white' and one may only give generalities as to teach emotion's association with individual chakras. Below are those that are accepted by most authorities. The 'Spiritual' links are purely objective and are based on anecdotal observation.

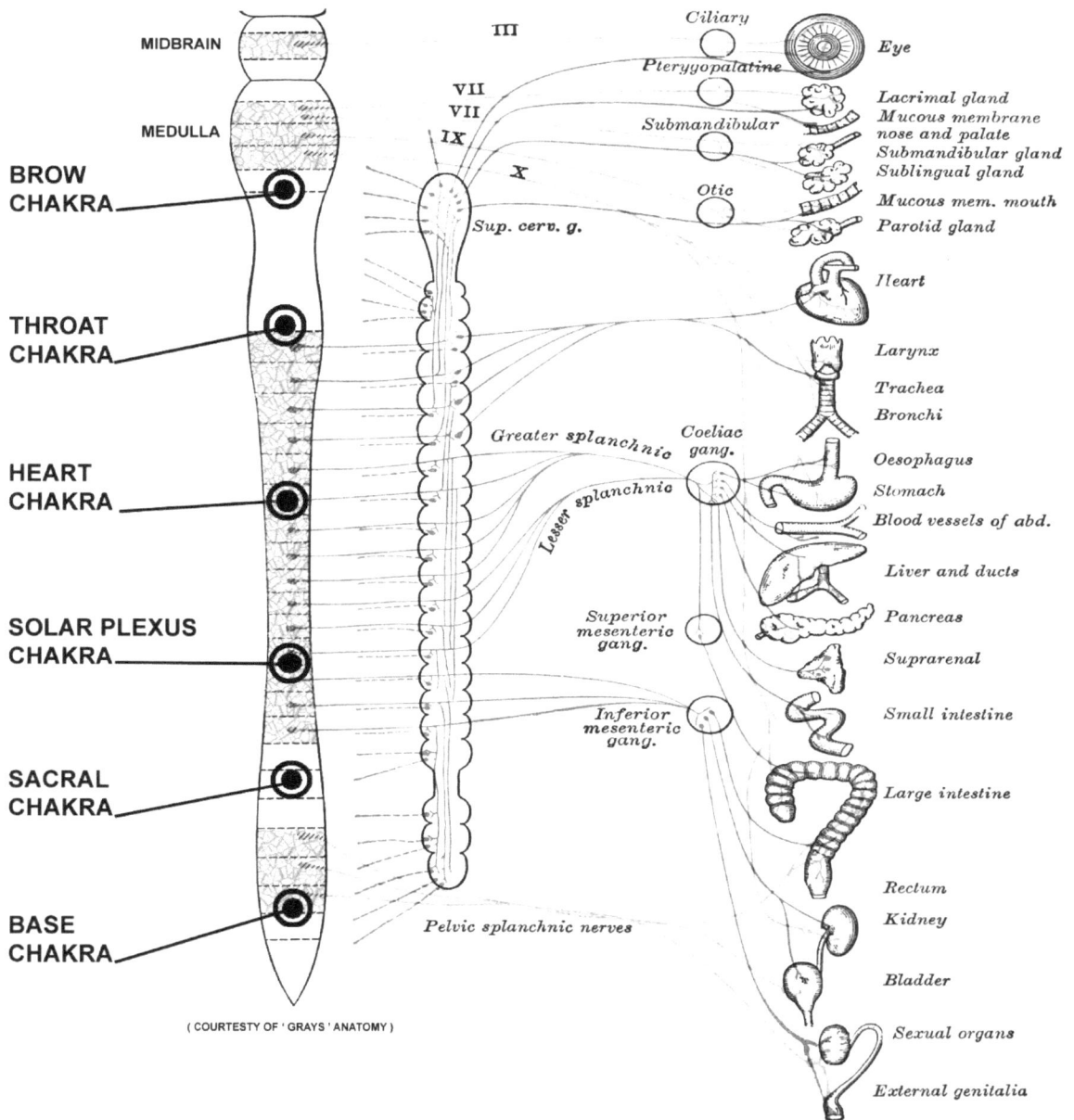

Figure 1.7.11 The ANS and the chakra energy system

- The CROWN chakra is linked with melancholia, highly strung and nervous, fidgety, head in the 'clouds', some phobias. ALL THAT IS
- The BROW chakra is linked with anger, rage, shyness, low confidence, highly strung, sleep disorders, lack of intuition, hallucinatory. INTUITION
- The THROAT chakra is linked with shyness, introvertness, paranoia, poor expression and communication, fear of speaking in public and fear of company. EXPRESSION
- The HEART chakra is linked with tearfulness, anxiety, affairs of the heart, inconsolable, cannot forgive others, excess empathy and compassion. LOVE

- The SOLAR PLEXUS chakra is linked with depression, worry, anxiety, low self-esteem, too much empathy. STABILIZING CONTROL
- The SACRAL chakra is linked with jealousy, envy, lust, low self-worth, nymphomania, tired all the time. PLEASURE AND ENJOYMENT
- The BASE chakra is linked with insecurity, doubt, many fears and phobias, not grounded, finance worries, dwells on materialism, overweight tendencies. MATERIALISM AND PHYSICAL

Associated Sound and Colours

Sound therapy and Colour therapy are very popular and seem to work very well, not only in isolation but also in combination with other approaches. Analysis and treatment can be enhanced when used with the chakras. Everyone has different sounds and colours that are both harmonizing and relaxing or jarring. In treatment mode, a sound or colour may be transmitted to a chakra either from a coloured lantern or Perspex, or by asking the patient to visualise a certain colour or sound or to recite mantras or affirmations. The harmonious resonating relationships to each chakra are as follows: -

- The CROWN chakra resonates to violet, gold, white and sound pitch B
- The BROW chakra resonates to indigo blue and sound pitch A
- The THROAT chakra resonates to turquoise, sky blue and sound pitch G
- The HEART chakra resonates to green and sound pitch F
- The SOLAR PLEXUS chakra resonates yellow and sound pitch E
- The SACRAL chakra resonates to orange and sound pitch D
- The BASE chakra resonates to red and sound pitch C

The practical chapters of Book Two will show how each of the vertebral and intervertebral levels may be influenced by one or more of the spinal chakras.

Chapter Eight - The Reflected Spine

Reflexology

As previously stated, reflexology is as old as the hills and has been around for as long as acupuncture and acupressure, having its roots within traditional Eastern medicine - along with diet, herbs and moxabustion. There are many traditional approaches to reflexology, heralding from India, China, Tibet, Korea and Japan, as well as some modern concepts. I personally see no difference between the two touch therapies of acupressure and reflexology. Each acupuncture point (acupoint) can be regarded as a reflected point (reflex) of an internal organ or system, and Auriculotherapy is synonymous with both acupuncture and reflexology. There are also scores of approaches to both acupressure and reflexology. When the word 'reflexology' is mentioned to the lay person, they immediately think of *foot* reflexology, but as all practitioners know, reflexes appear all over the body - including those of the spine.

What is a Reflex?

When this question is asked to delegates at the start of a workshop, heads would lower! Each person assumes that someone else would come up with a brilliant answer. Could it be a trick question? What is he getting at? Some folk would consider a reflex to be a nerve ending, others would say that it is a crystalline deposit of uric acid and calcium that builds up in the tissues when an internal organ is in a state of imbalance. Yet others would say that it is part of the meridian system of TCM or a hologram. I would say that a reflex is all of these things – and more. The word *reflex* is a shortened form of the word *reflected* and is therefore a reflected point, area or pathway of an internal organ, joint, bone, muscle or any part of the body that is telescoped or copied onto another part of the body. When the body suffers imbalance, sickness or dis-ease, this situation is mirrored or *reflected* to one or several other regions of the body that may be felt as tender areas or points. The only region of the body that will not exhibit tenderness, but acts purely as an analytical or diagnostic tool is the eye – as in iris diagnosis. The scientific community often scoff at the idea of reflexes and reflected pathways, merely because they haven't been scientifically proven to their satisfaction. How is it that the liver, for example, may be reflected onto the sole of the foot, the web between the great toe and second toe, the hand, tongue, eye, ear, abdomen, bowel, face, skull and radial pulse? I shall attempt a simplistic answer, because at heart I am a simple soul! The moment that each of us were conceived (conception) by an utter miracle of nature, that I like to call the Divine Spark, we were a combination of just two cells. At that moment, every part of our future bodies was encapsulated together in cells no larger than a pinhead. Then, as we start to grow in utero, an energetic link with every part of the body is maintained. We are each of us 'fearfully and wonderfully made' and each part of the body is in the exact position it should be to carry out its function. It is the same on the reflected body – each reflex of the body mirrors the exact position of the original. The stomach and solar plexus region of the body is roughly the centre of the body, and this is mirrored in the various reflected areas. You will find the stomach/ solar plexus reflex in the centre of the tongue, pulse, iris, arm, leg, hand, foot. The spine, that lies on the central vertical plane of the body, is mirrored or reflected on the central vertical planes of many parts of the body. The skull and head is obviously at the top of the body, and it is mirrored in a myriad of reflected regions, usually in an isolated position at the end of a limb, finger, toe etc. Although I find the practice of reflexology to be a fascinating discipline, I am more intrigued by the various placements on the body of the reflexes and the intrigue of energetically linking the reflex with the 'mother region' through either reflexology or acupressure.

Reflected areas of the Spine

The spine is reflected on the skull, temple, eye (iris), ear, tongue, arm, leg, foot and hand as well as the spine itself. These observations are based mostly on the several approaches of traditional reflexology including Chinese, Tibetan, Ayurvedic and Korean reflexology and the more modern philosophy of Applied Kinesiology. Anomalies often occur between one philosophy and another with the various reflex placements and there are several overlaps in placements between the various philosophies. This really confuses the reflexology student. They expect there to be one single definitive chart showing exactly where all the reflexes are – sadly this is not the case, and there are as many interpretations as there are folk who have pioneered these charts and given their names to them. [PS -I have pioneered many charts but couldn't give my name to them as they would sound 'angry' – *think about it*.]

The Foot

The foot represents the most common area of known reflexes and the one that is, by far, the most popular in utilising the placement of the reflexes into a practical therapy. Figure 1.8.1 shows a typical chart of foot reflexes on the plantar aspect.

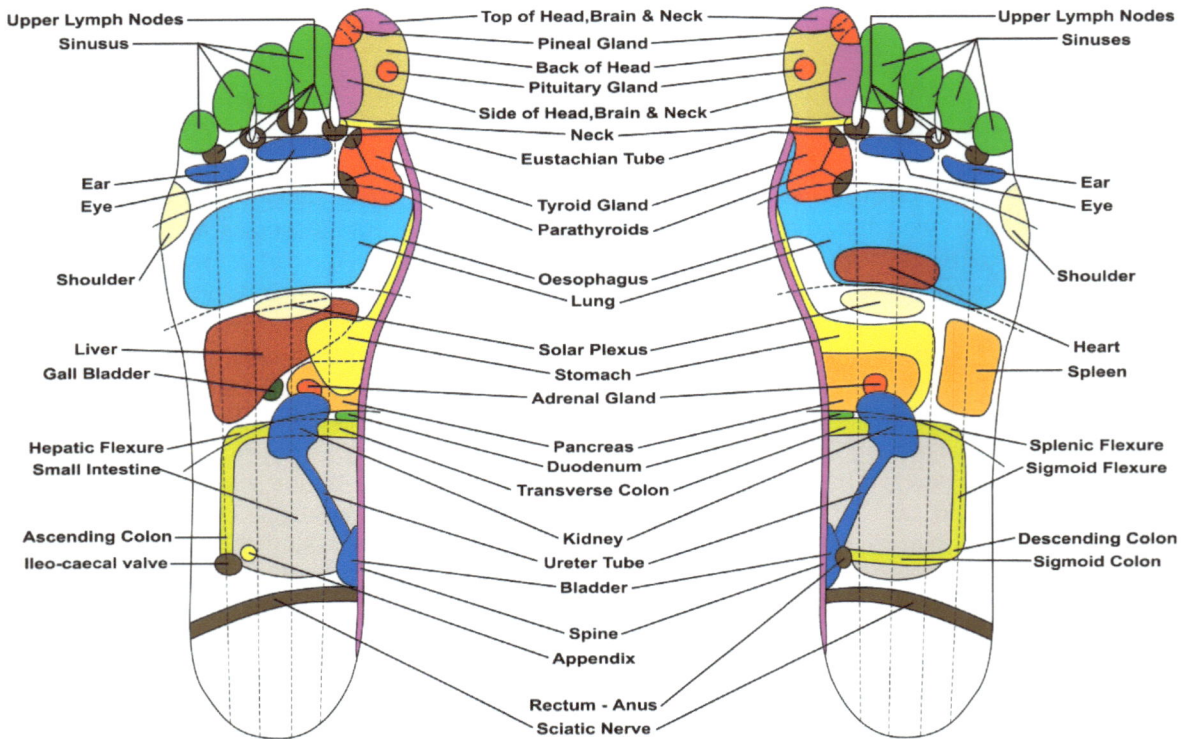

Upper Lymph Nodes
Sinusus
Ear
Eye
Shoulder
Liver
Gall Bladder
Hepatic Flexure
Small Intestine
Ascending Colon
Ileo-caecal valve

Top of Head,Brain & Neck
Pineal Gland
Back of Head
Pituitary Gland
Side of Head,Brain & Neck
Neck
Eustachian Tube
Tyroid Gland
Parathyroids
Oesophagus
Lung
Solar Plexus
Stomach
Adrenal Gland
Pancreas
Duodenum
Transverse Colon
Kidney
Ureter Tube
Bladder
Spine
Appendix
Rectum - Anus
Sciatic Nerve

Upper Lymph Nodes
Sinuses
Ear
Eye
Shoulder
Heart
Spleen
Splenic Flexure
Sigmoid Flexure
Descending Colon
Sigmoid Colon

Figure 1.8.1 Typical Foot Reflexology Chart – Plantar Aspect

The spine is reflected on the medial aspect, that is highlighted in Figures 1.8.2 and 1.8.3 and the skull/head is reflected in the great toe (details later in this section)

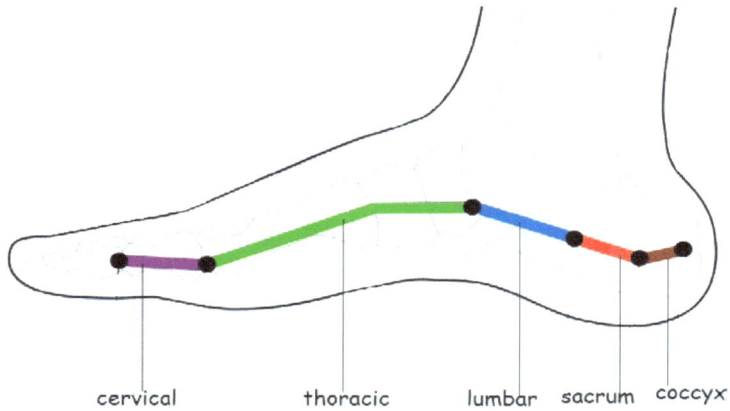

Figure 1.8.2 The Spine reflected in the Foot - Medial Aspect

Figure 1.8.2 above shows the spine reflected on the medial aspect of the foot. It is essentially down the central vertical axis as when the two feet are placed together, the spine is reflected down the middle. Figure 1.8.3 shows a more literal view of the spinal reflex.

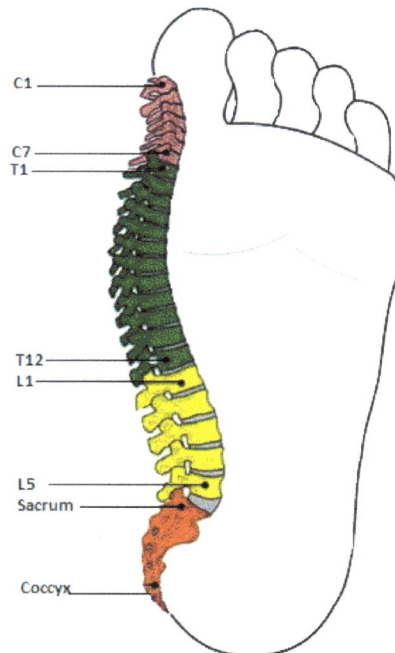

Figure 1.8.3 Spine reflected in the Spine – literal view (plantar aspect)

The following should be noted: -

1. The spine is positioned at the medial aspect of each foot with the spinous processes on the very medial aspect and the vertebral bodies and disc spaces slightly more lateral.

2. The individual levels of the spine are positioned exactly where they should be per the spinal anatomy i.e. the coccyx in the very lowest region and cervical at the inferior medial aspect of the great toe.

3. Pain and other forms of imbalance of the spine are mirrored in the reflex i.e. cervical pain will give discomfort in varying degrees at the cervical reflex region. When the spinal condition becomes chronic, such as osteoarthritis, soft tissue changes will sometimes occur at the reflex. A good example of this is the conditions of cervical spondylosis or chronic disc prolapse at the lower cervical will produce soft tissue and bony alterations around the head of the first metatarsal resulting in a bunion or osteo-arthritis of the metatarso-phalangeal joint

4. A chronic lower lumbar or sacral condition is mirrored at the lower medial aspect of the foot giving discomfort, circulatory and lymphatic changes and skin soreness.

5. The foot reflexes may be used in analytical or treatment mode.

The Hand

Hand reflexology has become very popular over the past twenty years or so. It is especially rewarding on clients who don't like their feet being touched and in teaching the client self-treatment that they can do at home – the hands, of course, are much easier to self-treat than the feet where dexterity and contortions are often required. Figure 1.8.4 shows typical arrangement of the reflexes on both plantar and dorsal aspects with the spine positioned on the medial aspect of the thumb. The cervical, thoracic, lumbar, sacrum and coccyx regions are positioned as you would expect per the spinal anatomy.

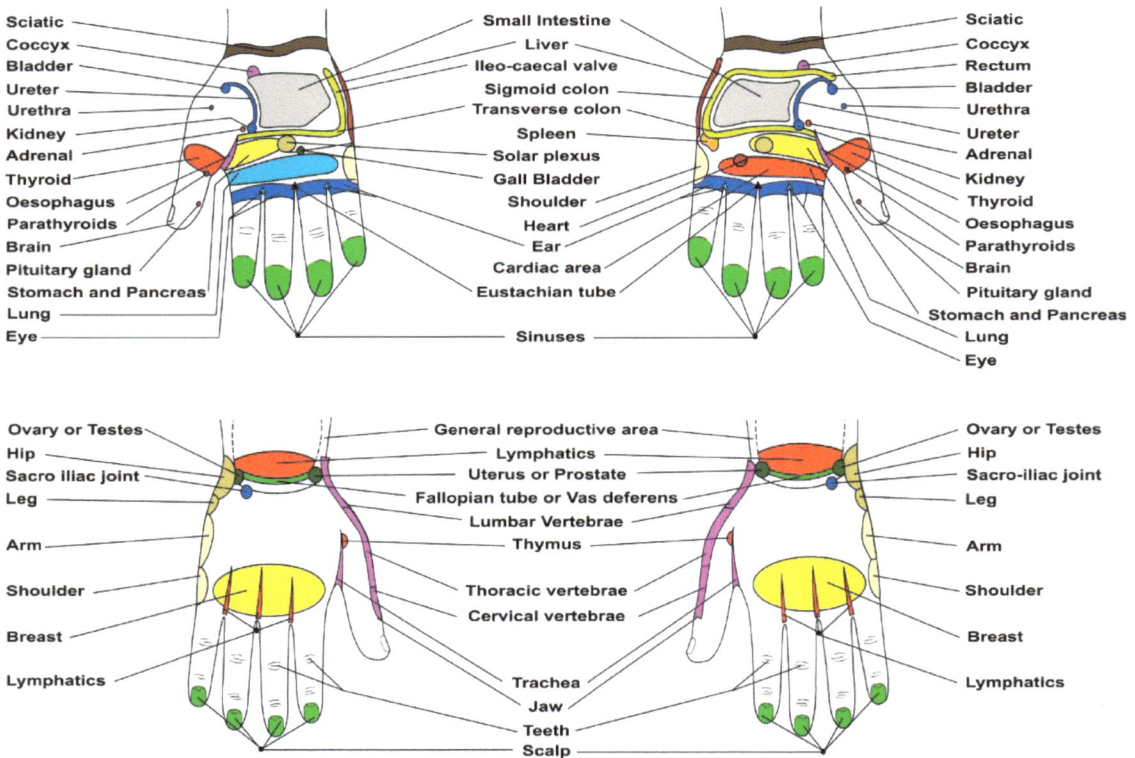

Figure 1.8.4 Typical Chart of Hand Reflexology – Dorsal and Plantar Aspect

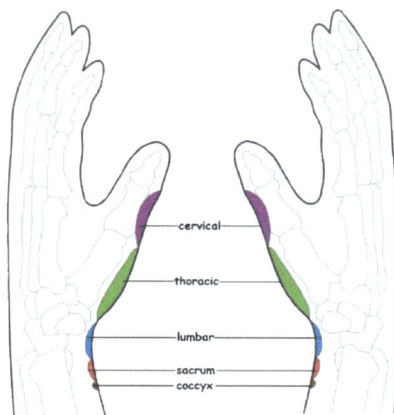

Figure 1.8.5 The Spine Reflected in the Hand

Figure 1.8.5 shows a different view of the spinal reflex. As the hands are mostly in the open and not 'hidden' and 'protected' like the feet, mirrored discomfort is much less in the hands, although it does occur and a trained reflexologist can illicit tenderness.

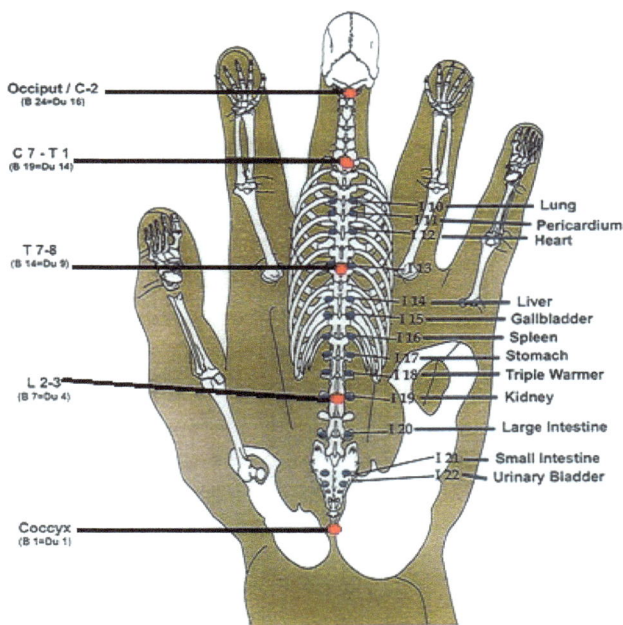

Figure 1.8.6 The Spine reflected in the Hand as per Korean Reflexology

Figure 1.8.6 shows a different concept of how the spine may be reflected in the hand. Korean reflexology has the spine reflected along the posterior aspect of the middle finger. Instead of placing the hands together and placing the spinal reflex where the thumbs meet, in Korean reflexology the spinal reflex is placed down the posterior aspect of just one hand. It is naturally placed down the centre of the middle finger with the skull at the tip of the middle finger and the various sections of the spinal column between it and the wrist joint. Note also that the limbs are also positioned on the dorsum of the hand, with the upper limbs on the ring and index fingers and the lower limbs on the thumb and little finger. The internal organs are positioned on the palmar aspect, as is the face.

The Arm and Leg

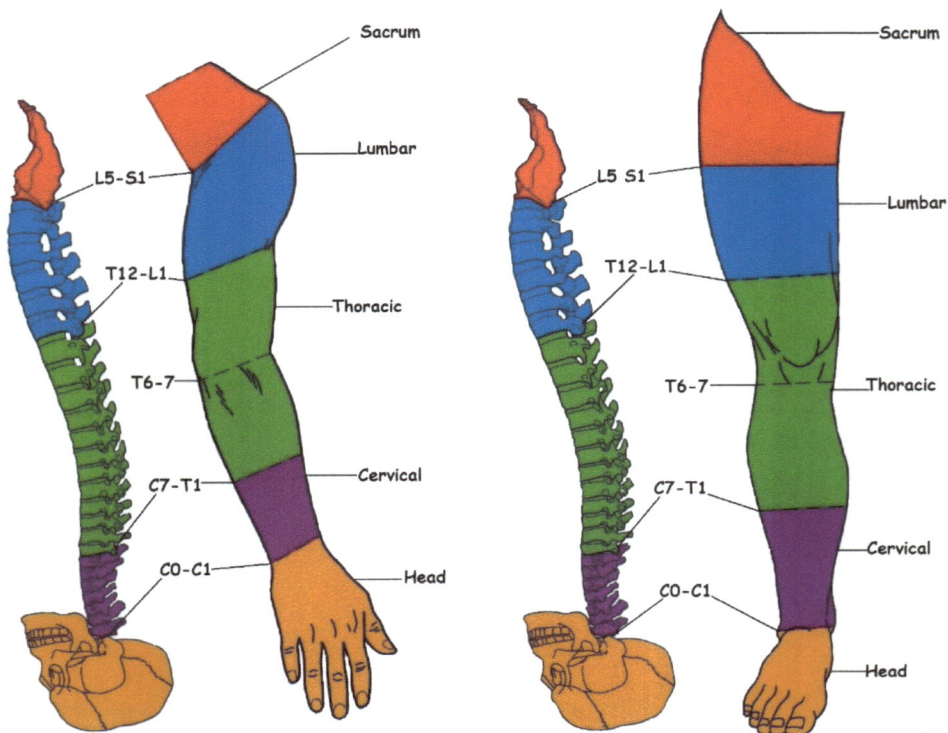

Figure 1.8.7 The Spine reflected in the Arm and Leg

The spine and skull are reflected in the arm and leg and may be used in both analysis and treatment.

- The head/skull is reflected in the whole of the foot or the whole of the hand. This contrasts with other concepts that shows the head/skull reflex covering the great toe and thumb – see section on skull reflexes.

- The occipito-atlas junction (C0-C1) is at the wrist and ankle joint

- The cervico-thoracic junction (C7-T1) is approximately half way up the forearm and lower leg

- The middle of the thoracic spine at T6-T7 is at the knee and elbow joint. Once again this shows the very middle of the spine reflected in the central part of the limb.

- The thoracic spine is reflected either side of the knee and elbow

- The thoraco-lumbar junction at T12-L1 is reflected half way down the leg and half way down the upper arm at the deltoid insertion.

- The lumbar spine is reflected around the upper leg to the groin and the upper arm to the shoulder.

- The lumbo-sacral junction at L5-S1 is reflected at the hip and shoulder joints

- The sacrum is reflected at the very top of the leg and medial aspect of the arm

I formulated the above illustration several years and it appears on my A1 poster 'The Holistic Spine – Associations and Reflections'. I then decided to take it one stage further in narrowing down exactly where each vertebra is reflected on the limbs. Figures 1.8.8 and 1.8.9 refer.

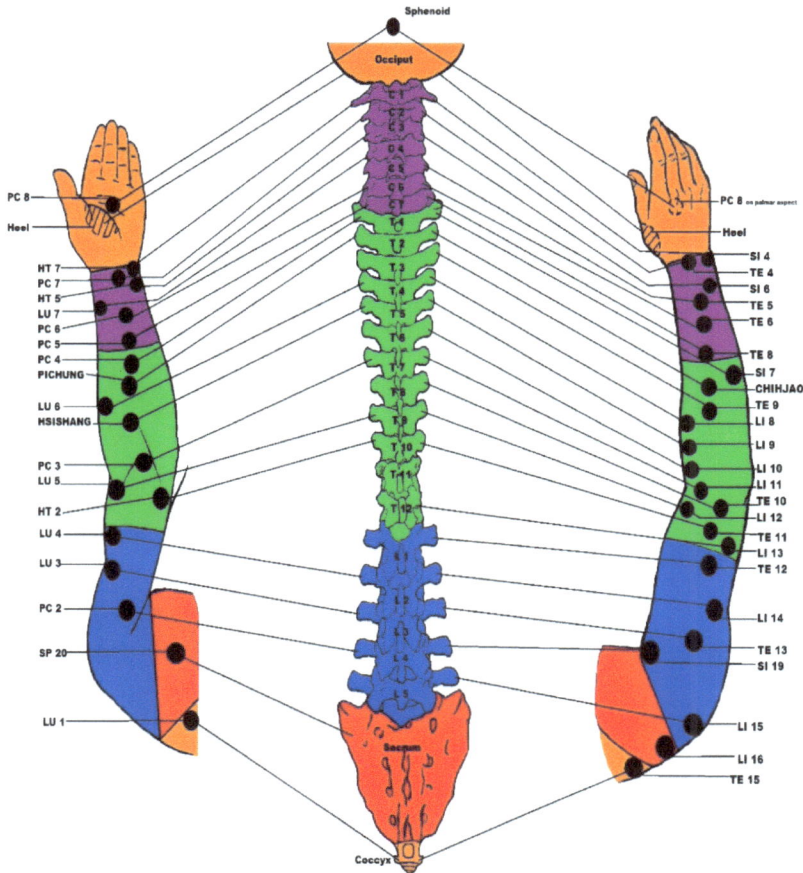

Figure 1.8.8 The Spine reflected at acupoints on the Arm

To save giving exact anatomical positions that can become confusing in their explanations, I decided to show how each vertebra is related to an individual acupuncture point. Although I pioneered these charts several years ago, and have taught them many times – it is the first time they have been published. Each of the arm/leg illustrations show the yin and yang acupoints for each of the vertebrae. Acupuncture points are, of course, reflected points of internal organs and systems and these charts give an indication which acupoint is related to each vertebra. This is useful knowledge in both analysis and treatment modes. In analytical mode, when you think a spinal problem is prevalent but are unsure as to the exact one – gently palpate the arm or leg to illicit tenderness. The client may also indicate areas of tenderness on the limbs. Tenderness on the 'yin' aspect indicates a chronic spinal imbalance, whereas tenderness on a 'yang' acupoint indicates an acute condition. As indicated previously, the more chronic the spinal condition, the more sluggish the tissues are around the reflected point.

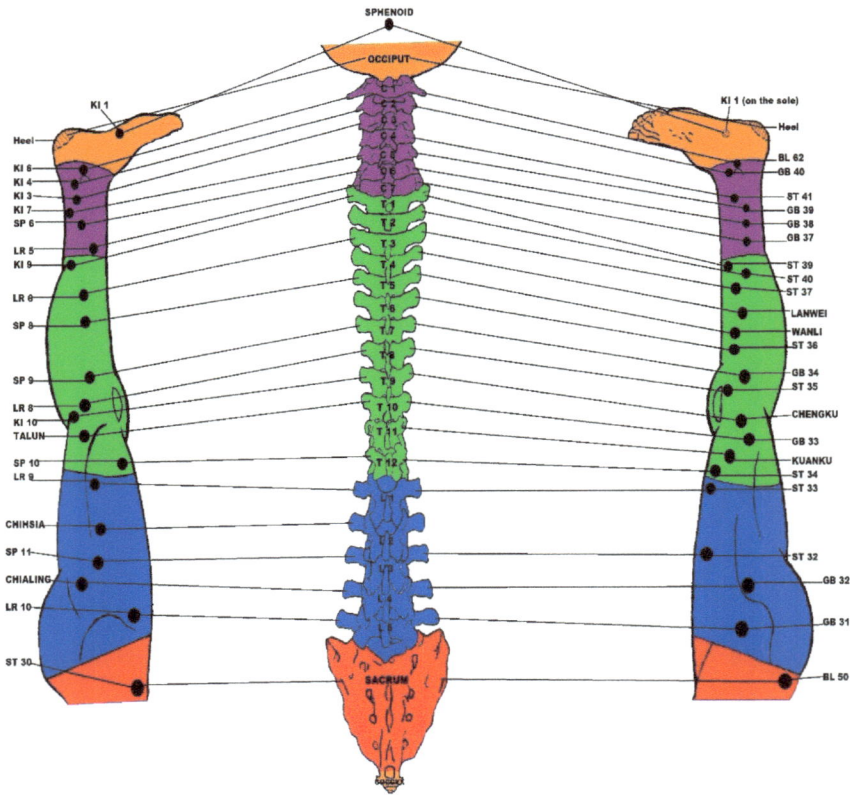

Figure 1.8.9 The Spine reflected at acupoints on the Leg

The use of the reflected spine on the arm/leg in treatment mode will be discussed in Book Two

The Head

We now proceed to the various areas on the head where the spine is reflected. These are extremely important regions in therapy and can be powerful tools in both assessment and treatment modes. The reflected points around the ear, face and skull are subtler than their hand/foot/arm/leg counterparts. Some practitioners steer away from working around the head as they feel 'all thumbs' and clumsy and some patients don't like this approach as it feels invasive. I was always fortunate in practice in that I had worked with craniosacral therapy as well as acupuncture, so was used to working around the head and able to detect the many nuances of touch associated with craniosacral therapy as well as cranial osteopathy. The golden rule with all therapy is to only practice that with which you are comfortable (and qualified in)

The Ear

The outer ear is a remarkable region of the body and can be extremely powerful when used with acupuncture, or touch therapy. It is said to be the outward expression of the hypothalamus region of the brain and is therefore used in treating emotional and mental imbalance as well as treating cravings as in smoking and drugs. Auriculotherapy is a post graduate study that may take several months to learn – but it is well worth it in that the knowledge will repay you time and time again in the treatment of many conditions. Figure 1.8.10 shows a typical outer ear with the body's reflexes superimposed.

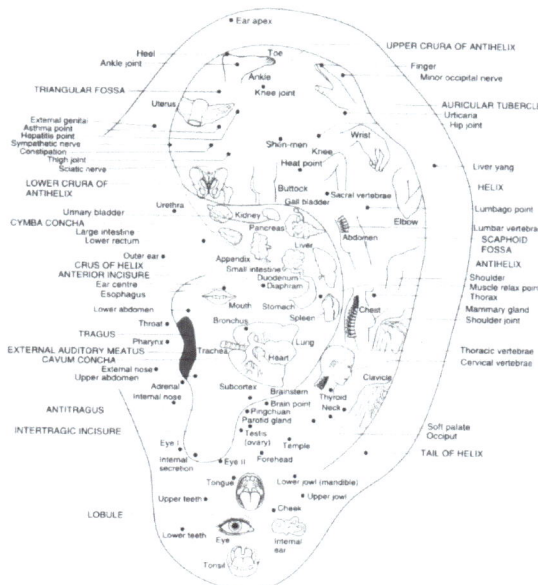

Figure 1.8.10 The Ear Reflexes as used in Auriculotherapy

The ear reflexes may be viewed as an upside-down foetus, with the head within the pinna (lobe), the internal organs (yin) protected on the medial aspect and the limbs (yang) on the lateral aspect. You will be able to ascertain the various aspects of the spine in the above illustration but this is made clearer in Figure 1.8.11 below shown in more diagrammatic form.

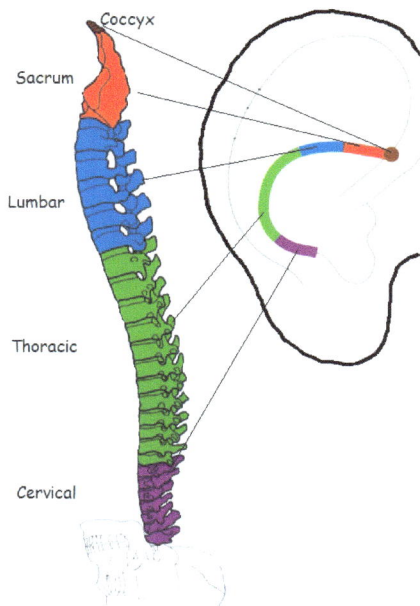

Figure 1.8.11 Diagrammatic interpretation of the Reflected Spine in the Ear

103

Palpation in analytical mode is very different to palpation on the rest of the body because of the size of the ear and the adjacency of the reflex points. A small metal probe, specifically engineered for the task, is used, with very little pressure to ascertain if a point is sensitive or painful. Never use a needle or sharp pointed instrument. A cotton bud may be used but this isn't very accurate. The ideal 'tool', of course, would be the finger, but it must be the little finger and, usually, there is very little sensitivity in this finger that is rarely used in any other form of acupressure/reflexology.

The Skull

There are two regions of spinal reflection on the skull – the mid line and the temple. Two cranial bones – the occiput and sphenoid are also reflected to the spine – details later.

The Skull- Midline

Figure 1.8.12 gives the position of the double aspected reflected spine along the midline aspect of the skull. Acupoint Gov 20 represents the centre between the two reflections.

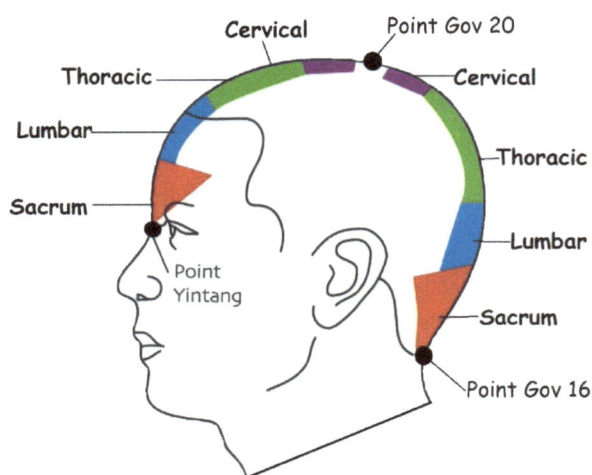

Figure 1.8.12 The Reflected Spine on the Skull – Midline

Gov 20 is situated on the central line exactly half way between the centre of the eyebrows (Yintang) and the base of the skull (Gov 16) in the midline and halfway between the anterior aspect of both ears in the sagittal plane. The cervical spine is reflected adjacent to Gov 20 and the sacrum is reflected on the forehead and on the occiput. The same rules apply to these reflected spinal aspects as with all the others, in that the reflected point will become tender or sensitive when that part of the spine is in a state of imbalance. This reflected area is very useful in treatment and analysis.

The Temporal Bone

The whole of the spine is reflected on the temporal bone (temple) at the lateral aspect of the skull in an area called the Temporo-Sphenoidal Line (TSL)– Figure 1.8.13 refers. The philosophy of the TSL dates to the pioneer days of the middle of the twentieth century and is accredited to Dr. George Goodheart and other pioneers of Applied Kinesiology. In those early chiropractic texts, it categorically stated that the TSL is used in analysis only and purely to ascertain the condition of a muscle, but I modified the original theory to include treatment benefits as well. Several points of acute tenderness may exist along the TSL. As stated these were associated with muscles that were in spasm, flaccid or some other form of imbalance. When I studied this phenomenon in the late 1970's I soon realised that the constant muscle testing that was associated with these points was extremely tedious and not my favourite occupation.

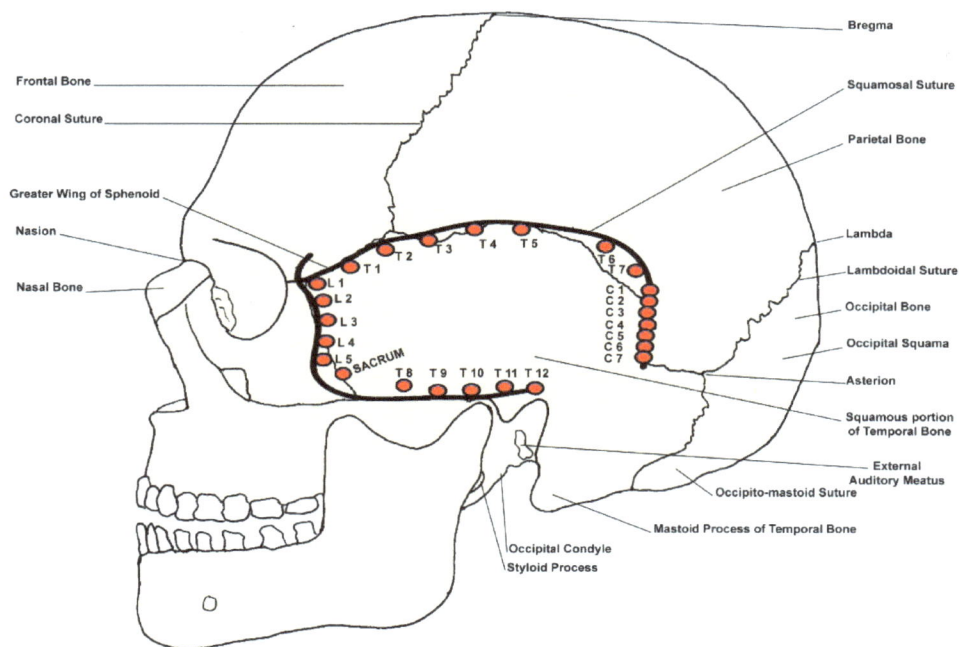

Figure 1.8.13 The Temporo-Sphenoidal Line (TSL)

I have discovered the TSL to be a powerful reflected region showing the vertebral levels as well. In analytical mode, the discomfort on gentle palpation shows imbalance in the corresponding vertebra – acute lesions showing more tenderness than chronic lesions. In treatment mode (expanded in Book Two), once the level of the spinal lesion is known, the relevant reflex is held either side for between one and five minutes. This affords relief of tension and discomfort at the vertebral level and paves the way for more intensive therapy using local treatment or other reflected points for the specific spinal level.

The spinal reflexes on the head are completed with two regions that are only used in analytical and assessment mode – the eye and tongue.

The Eye (Iris)

Iris Diagnosis (Iridology) represents a fascinating study and one that can take several years to perfect. In common with the other reflected regions, the centre of the iris represents the centre of the body and the outside represents the exterior. The area just around the pupil represents the stomach and the outside of the ring represents the skin. Any irregularity with any organ, such as allergic syndromes or inflammation shows up yellow or orange in the form of a corona. The remainder of the iris represents the remainder of the body that many be easily identified by looking at the relevant positions of the hands of the clock. Brown, blue, black or grey markings in the exact area corresponding to an individual body part signifies some state of imbalance in that region of the body. The spots appear almost immediately that the lesion occurs and disappears almost as quickly once the lesion has been correctly treated. The spinal reflexes appear on the lower medial aspects of each eye with the coccyx almost on the exterior aspect at 20 past the hour on the clock and the upper cervical region closer to the centre on the 15 minutes past the hour. The coloured changes in the iris are best detected with a special magnifying glass. Iridology represents a superb way of assessing any condition. The more chronic the condition, the darker the colour in the iris. Figure 1.8.14 shows the iris reflexes.

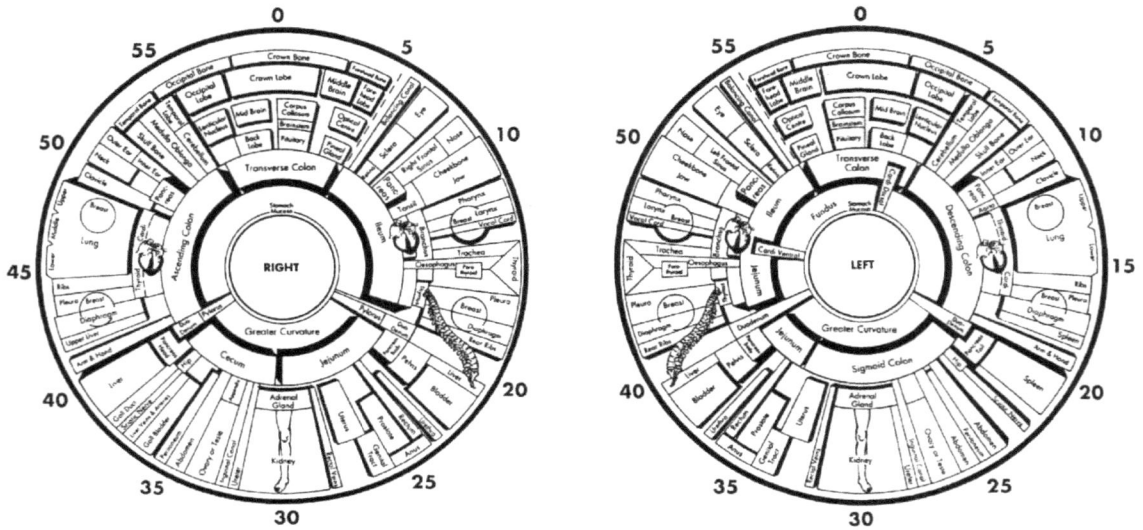

Figure 1.8.14 Iris Diagnosis (Iridology)

The Tongue

Tongue diagnosis stems directly from traditional Chinese medicine and was a major player for centuries. The skills required for doing tongue diagnosis appear to have been lost in this modern era of acupuncture practice – such a pity! As with every other reflected region, the centre of the reflected area represents the centre of the body i.e. stomach. In modern western medicine, the tongue represents the outward expression of the stomach and any imbalance can be detected there. The kidney/bladder regions are reflected at the root of the tongue, the heart and pericardium at the tip, the lungs on the right middle side and the liver/gall bladder on the left middle region. Figure 1.8.15 shows a typical diagrammatic representation of the reflected organs – the colour coding is that of the Law of Five Transformations (Elements). The great beauty of tongue diagnosis is that changes appear in the tongue before symptoms appear in the body. Tongue diagnosis, combined with pulse and abdominal diagnosis are the cornerstones of traditional diagnosis in Chinese medicine. This, of course, is a far cry from the 'symptomatic pin pricking' that occurs in modern medical acupuncture.

I was very fortunate in that I was a traditional acupuncturist as well as a chartered physiotherapist. With each chronic soft tissue and spinal condition patient that I saw, I observed that chronic spinal conditions were reflected to all the regions (that have been mentioned) as well as on the tongue. This started when I noticed that many of my lumbar spine arthritis patients also had certain changes in the root of the tongue – such as discolouration, papule formation or inflammation. Similarly, the chronic mid dorsal patients had mid tongue changes and cervical had tip of tongue alterations. The more chronic the spinal condition - the darker the tongue regions. Figure 1.8.16 refers

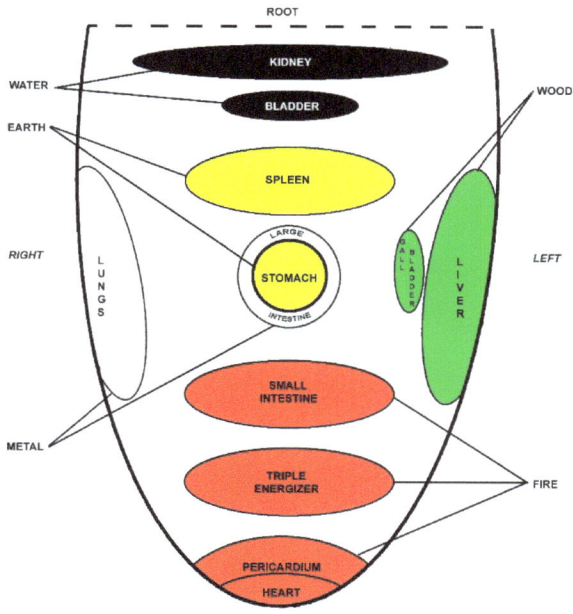

Figure 1.8.15 Tongue Diagnosis Regions of TCM

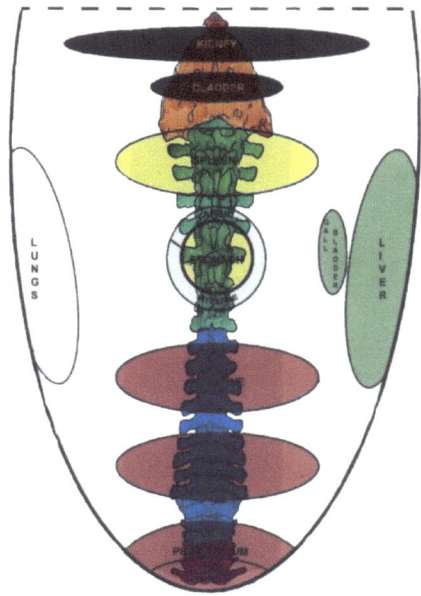

Figure 1.8.16 Reflected Spine superimposed on the Tongue

The Spine

Although not strictly coming under the heading of reflexology and the reflection of the spine on other parts of the body, it can be said that the spine is reflected on itself. Four major concepts are included in this category – the 'Lovett Brother', Sacro-Occipital Technique, Cranio-Sacral Reflexology and Cranio-Sacral Reflextherapy. The last two will be discussed in Book Two.

Lovett Brother

The concept of the Lovett Brother has been accepted in the chiropractic world for over a century. It is based on the work of Robert W. Lovett who, in 1913, wrote a book called 'Lateral Curvature of the Spine and Round Shoulders' – published by Blakiston's in Philadelphia. The theory is that each vertebra is coupled with another vertebra and when one is affected by injury, misalignment or other changes, the coupled vertebra is also affected. As you can see from the Figure 1.8.17 it is a question of 'as above – so below'.

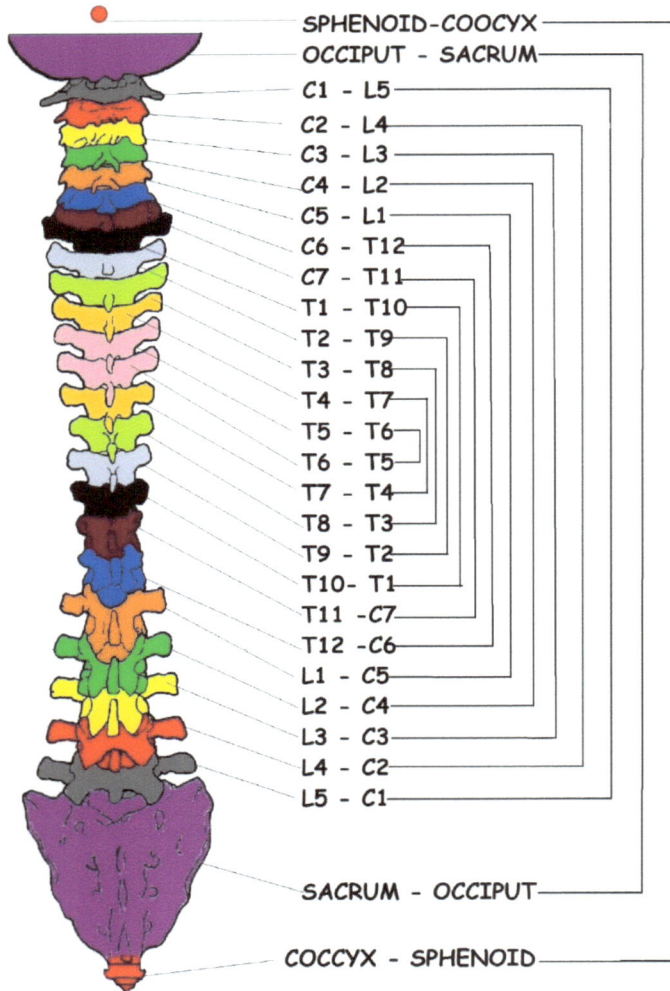

Figure 1.8.17 Interpretation of the Lovett Brother

It is said that the spine 'pivots' around its centre i.e. T5-T6 and the vertebra above is coupled with the vertebra below. Therefore, T4 is coupled with T7, T3 with T8 and so on. At the extremities, one can see that the Sphenoid is coupled with the Coccyx, the Occiput with the Sacrum and the Atlas with L5. In chiropractic terms, it is said that the coupled vertebra is misplaced either in the same plane or the opposite plane. My research into this concept has shown that when there is pain and soft tissue congestion around an individual vertebra, this is reflected to its coupled vertebra that also exhibits pain and discomfort. This does not occur immediately after the trauma but certainly within a couple of weeks if treatment of the lesion isn't successfully completed. This concept is also borne out of another idea of Sacro-Occipital Therapy which couples the vertebral levels in a similar way.

Sacro-Occipital Technique

Another type of vertebral adjustment and 'balancing' is known as Sacro-Occipital Technique (SOT). The Sacro-Occipital Technique, a major player in chiropractic technique, was developed by osteopath and chiropractor Major Bertrand DeJarnette in the 1920's. The technique is based on normalising the relationship between the extremities of the spinal column.

The Sacro-Occipital Technique itself is performed by analysing the condition of the patient's spine in three positions – vertical, prone, and supine. The SOT practitioner then analyses the nerve health and flow of cerebro-spinal fluid from the brain to the spine, and adjusts vertebrae to improve this flow. During this process, he/she may palpate the skull to adjust the cranial bones, while simultaneously massaging or "pumping" various vertebrae to remove blockages that could interfere with cerebro-spinal fluid flow. The SOT practitioner often uses the weight of the patient's own body to correct abnormalities in the body. For example, treatment may involve placing wedge-shaped foam cushions under certain parts of the body to realign the pelvis as the patient reclines on them.

Like other chiropractic techniques, SOT seeks to correct abnormalities in the spine that produce back, arm, leg or head pain. Patients suffering from migraine, neck and shoulder pain, fatigue and nervous disorders can benefit immediately from Sacro-Occipital manipulation. However, the main goal of a chiropractic SOT treatment is not to eliminate or reduce pain, it is to normalise the function of the brain and spinal cord. SOT seeks to improve the overall transmission of nerve impulses from the brain down the spine and to other areas of the body. Equal emphasis is placed in SOT treatment on the proper positioning of the pelvis. The spine and skull, shoulders and arms are supported above the pelvis, and the legs and feet are supported below. Thus, an improperly aligned pelvis can cause postural irregularities, problems with normal functioning of the skull and jaw, and muscular dysfunction. As the name sacro-occipital implies, SOT treatment focuses on both ends of the spine, because they are so interrelated. By correcting imbalances both in the skull and in the pelvis, communication is improved along the entire spinal column.

Self-help SOT

This is a very simple technique that patients can perform on themselves. They are asked to adopt the supine lying position with the body as stretched out as possible i.e. best done lying on a bed, not on a settee. Place the palm of one hand under the occiput and gently rest the skull on the hand. Place the back of the other hand under the sacrum and allow the body to relax, as far as is able, into this posture for as long as able before the advent of 'pins and needles' in the arms. What is noticeable, after just a minute or so, is that the anterior aspect of the torso, especially the stomach, seems to relax. This may be followed by a deep breath or sigh. This shows that the sympathetic nervous system is relaxing. Visualizations will help to augment the session, as will mediation or silent mantras. The patient may be instructed to imaging having a 'long and unwound' spinal column, or to relaxing the erector spinae muscles. They could also concentrate on just one aspect of the spine 'unwinding' or the whole of the spine – each person is different. Having practiced this technique myself for many years, I can thoroughly recommend its efficacy.

The Posterior Reflexes

The Posterior Reflexes are reflected regions of internal organs on the back (not strictly on the spine). They are the back's equivalent of abdominal reflexes. They may be used in both analysis and treatment and are very useful in acute conditions. The colour coding indicates their Five Element relationship. The spinal ones tend to coincide with the Back-Transporting Points Figure 1.8.18 refers

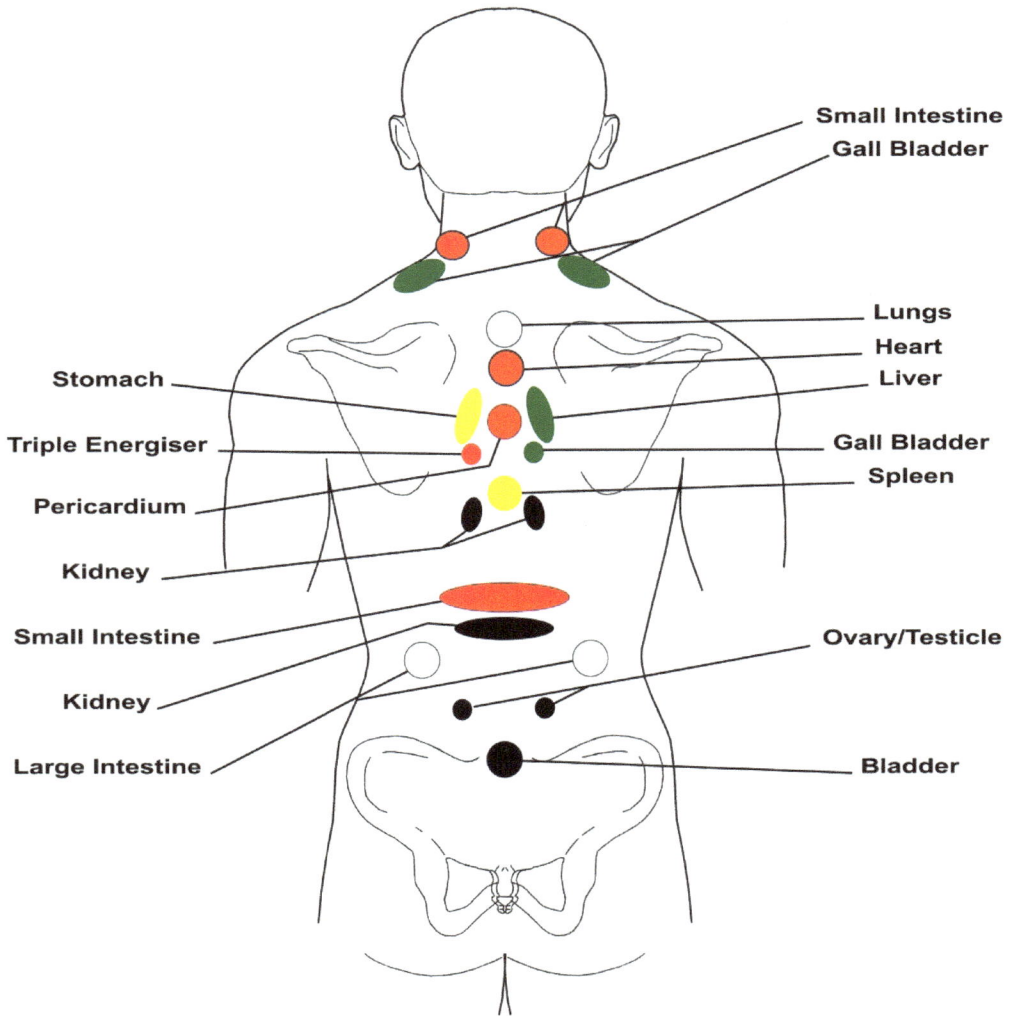

Figure 1.8.18 The Posterior Reflexes

Small Intestine
Gall Bladder

Lungs
Heart
Liver

Stomach

Gall Bladder
Spleen

Triple Energiser

Pericardium

Kidney

Small Intestine

Ovary/Testicle

Kidney

Large Intestine

Bladder

CHAPTER NINE
PERSONALITY TRAITS REFLECTED ON THE SPINE

The last chapter of Part One of this book discussed how the tissues connected with the spine could be influenced by our mental processes and emotions. This chapter discusses how the spine and each of the various segmental levels can be influenced by our 'character and personality'. Sounds farfetched? Yes, I know it does, and it certainly cannot be tested scientifically, but I have the anecdotal evidence of my own spinal patients and the hundreds of practitioners who have contacted me to verify my work.

During my long career, I have had the privilege of meeting some remarkable people who have been (and still are) pioneers in their own field. Such a person is Christine (Chris) Stormer-Fryer. Chris was born in Nairobi, Kenya before moving to the UK where she trained and worked as a nurse. She then emigrated to South Africa and still lives there with her husband John, where they run Soul Retreats and safaris. I met Chris in 1995 when she visited the UK to give some seminars on universal reflexology. I trained in her version of reflexology and the 'Language of the Feet'. The latter is a masterpiece and I would advise any of my reflexology readers to purchase a copy – it will open your eyes.

Language of the Feet
This concept deals with the general analysis of a client just by observing the feet. Chris calls it 'feetspeak'. It deals with the fact that the feet, in all its myriad parts is a reflected area of the rest of the body, and the marks of life's experiences impress the soul and soles, and are reflected on the feet long before being mirrored in the rest of the body as symptoms. Understanding these reflections allows for early detection of dis-ease and prevents inner turmoil before damage occurs on all levels. Although, in her book, all aspects of the feet are discussed, I shall cover the 5 zones i.e. the five toes and vertical extensions to the heel, and their significance towards understanding a person's character and personality.

- Big toe -often called the Great toe – is the **Thinking** toe that also deals with **Intuition**. In general reflexology, the great toe, naturally represents the head and the medial aspect of the upper spine as well as the central nervous system, sinuses. The lower part of this vertical zone deals with the remainder of the spine. This zone symbolizes intellectual thought, intuition and spirituality.

- Second toe – is the **Feeling** toe that also deals with **Emotions**. It symbolizes thoughts regarding personal perceptions of the self. It is linked with the heart, lungs, breasts, thyroid gland and solar plexus

- Third toe – is the **Doing** toe that also deals with **Action**. It symbolizes self-empowerment and instinctive survival. It is linked to the digestive system, liver, gall bladder, stomach, pancreas, adrenal glands and solar plexus.

- Fourth toe – is the **Communications** toe that deals also with **Relationships**. It symbolizes pleasurable thoughts that enhance relationships and communication. It is linked to the circulatory, lymphatic and excretory systems

- Little toe – is **Family, Security** and **Movement** toe. It is linked to the skeletal and muscular systems.

There is obviously a great deal more information that you may ascertain from the condition of each of the toes, but the above is a flavour. Simply put, the toe and related region reflects the person's personality archetype in its shape, size, irregularity etc. When holistic reflexology is carried out just using the zones, the toe improves as well as the body part and emotion to which it is a reflected region.

The Personality Traits transposed to the Feet

I proceeded to take Chris's work as a template and divide the feet into five vertical and five horizontal zones, each giving the character/personality previously described. This work was also based on the zones theory of reflexology – described earlier in this Part. Figure 1.9.1 shows my first effort as an illustration. I proceeded to divide each of the regions into a further five (not shown). This was to become significant when all this was transposed to the spine. I also used Chris's original colour coding, that was remarkably like the typical chakra colours.

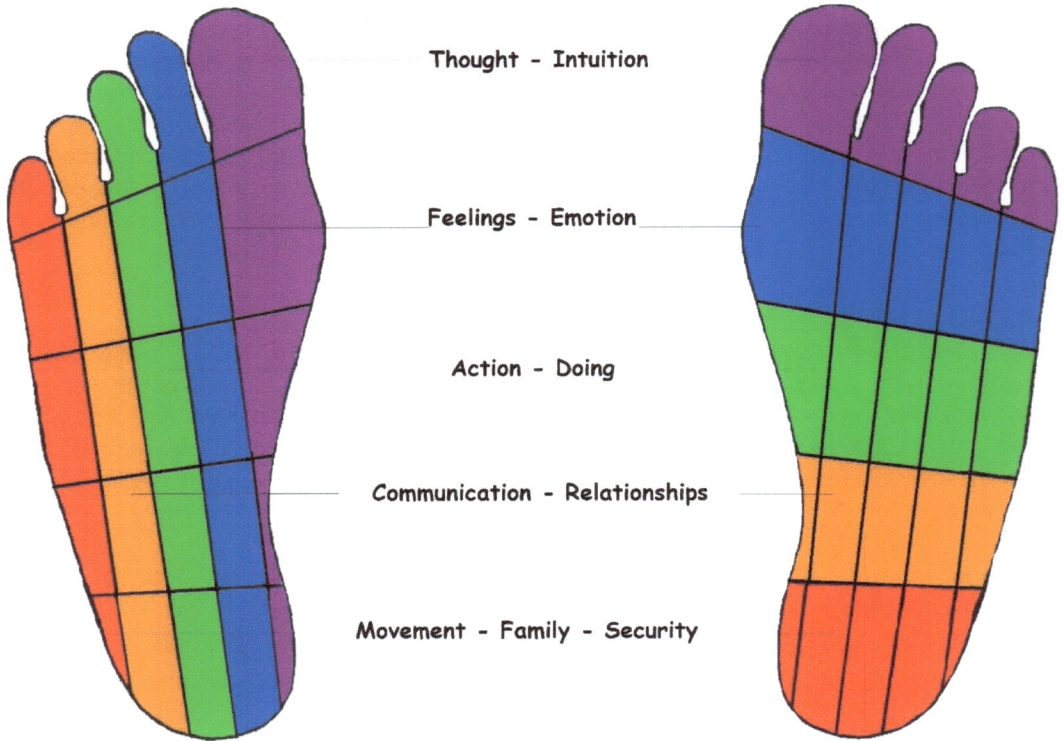

Thought - Intuition

Feelings - Emotion

Action - Doing

Communication - Relationships

Movement - Family - Security

Figure 1.9.1 The five vertical and horizontal zones on the feet

I now saw my reflexology clients in a new light, and treated only on the zones, after establishing what 'archetypes' they were at consultation. I also practised Metamorphic Technique then, which totally complemented this approach of treatment. I was finding that, with very few exceptions, it didn't matter what physical conditions and symptoms the patient had, when treating them on a purely 'etheric and emotional' level, the physical symptoms were helped alongside the emotional ones.

The Personality Traits transposed to the Body

I wasn't just practising reflexology then, so wearing my physiotherapist hat, I slowly transposed the zones on to the rest of the body. This proved easier than I thought it would do and the various regions together with their personality traits quickly fell into place. These, eventually became the genesis of my work with the minor chakras and pain relief. Figure 1.9.2 shows my early attempts at transposing the five zones on to the body. I am only showing the horizontal regions, but it is possible to use this work with the five vertical zones (but it isn't as easy).

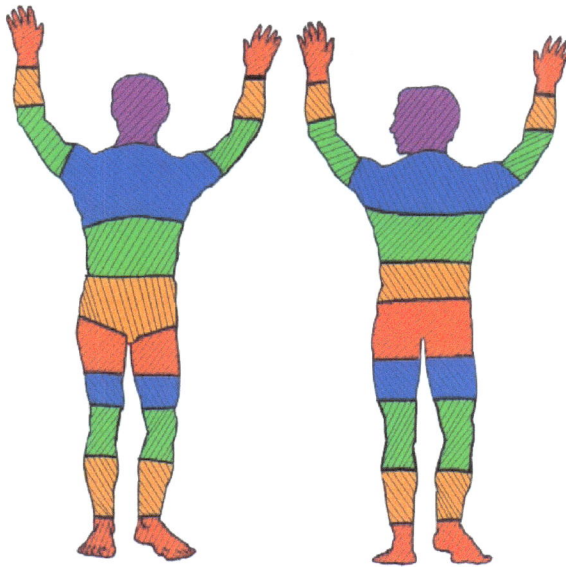

🟪	Thought - Intuition
🟦	Feelings - Emotion
🟩	Action - Doing
🟧	Communication - Relationships
🟥	Movement - Family - Security

Figure 1.9.2 The five horizontal zones on the body

The Personality Traits transposed on to the Spine

As I was interested in all things spinal, I proceeded to transpose the personality zones to the different regions of the spine. This took me some time to do (life in general gets in the way of progress) and the finished product is shown in Figure 1.9.3. When it was completed, I was astonished how accurate it was when viewing my patients with this new-found information. The rationale was as follows: -

- The coccyx – i.e. the base of the spine or the 'foundations of the building' is linked to our ability to move freely without constraint. Family worries and general security are also linked with this very important aspect of the spine. Symptomatically, when family or security worries are highlighted for some time, this gives rise to lower sacral stiffness, coccyx pain, bladder irritation and general stiffness of the spine. You will see in Book Two how important to the mobility of the rest of the spine the coccyx is.

- The sacrum, sacroiliac joints and hip joints are linked with communication and relationships. It is the 'sexual' aspect of the body. When libido is low, there is often stiffness around this region.

- The lower thoracic and lumbar spine are linked with action and doing. This region has the largest vertebrae and takes most of the body weight, so when fully energised there is maximum movement and action. The opposite is where action and potential are limited. This may cause lower spinal pain and stiffness as well as related internal organ (bowel) imbalance.

- The lower cervical and the thoracic spine to T9 are linked with our feelings and emotions. This region is linked with the heart, lungs and other internal organs. It is also the region that houses most of the sympathetic nerves that become agitated with stress situations

- The upper three cervical vertebrae are related with our thoughts and intuition. In Ayurvedic medicine this region is related to the Third Eye (Ajna) chakra that deals with our intuition and foresight. When this becomes 'blocked' or congested it gives rise to symptoms such as headache or migraine.

- The occiput is related (as is the coccyx) with movement, family and security – as above, so below.

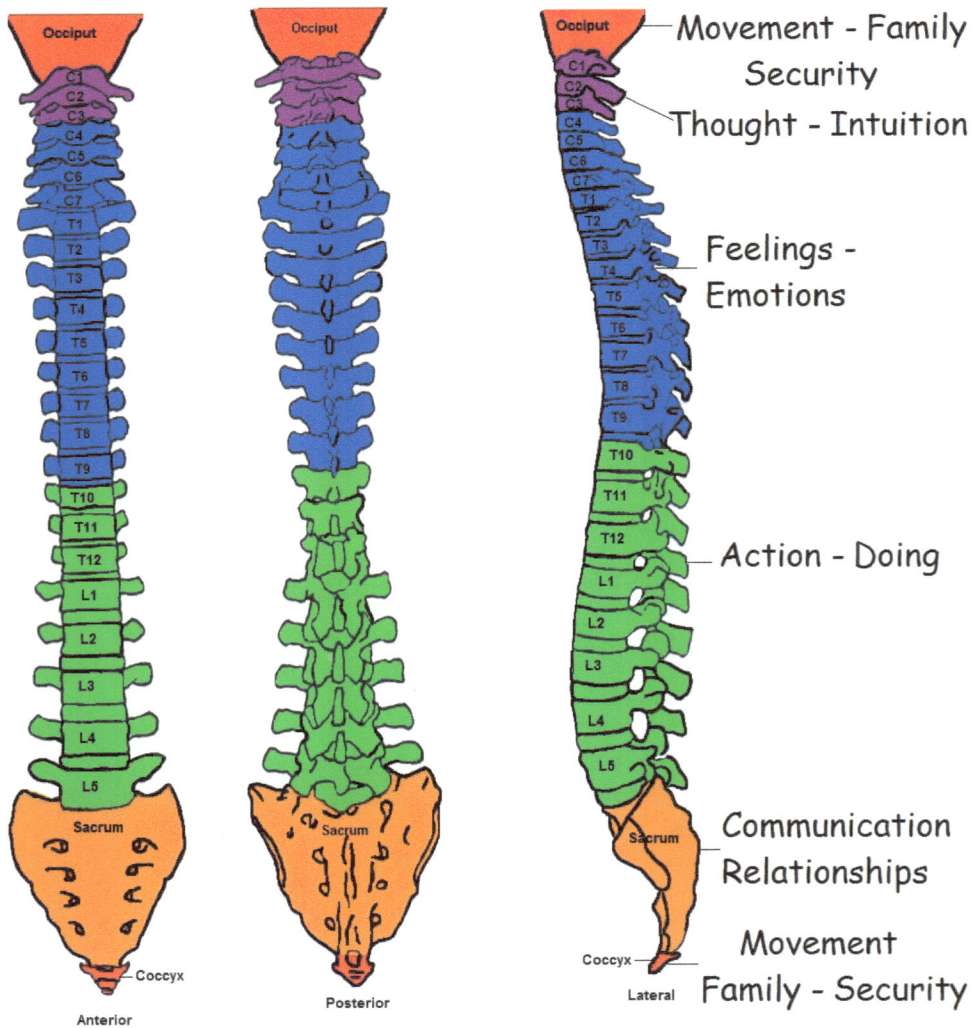

Figure 1.9.3 Personality traits transposed to the spine (general)

I then revisited Chris's original foot zones to find that each of the main zones were divided into a further five (horizontal and vertical) when the minutia of individual reflexes may be felt and treated in the feet (or

114

hand). I then decided to see if individual vertebrae or sets of adjacent vertebrae could be linked to the personality traits. This proved to be quite difficult to do, but when completed I realised that each seemed to be correct. I did this work using a combination of Chris's work, Polarity therapy and my own work with the chakra energy system. The final product is shown in Figure 1.9.4. I shall not, here, explain the rationale behind each one as this will be discussed in detail in the first part of Book Two.

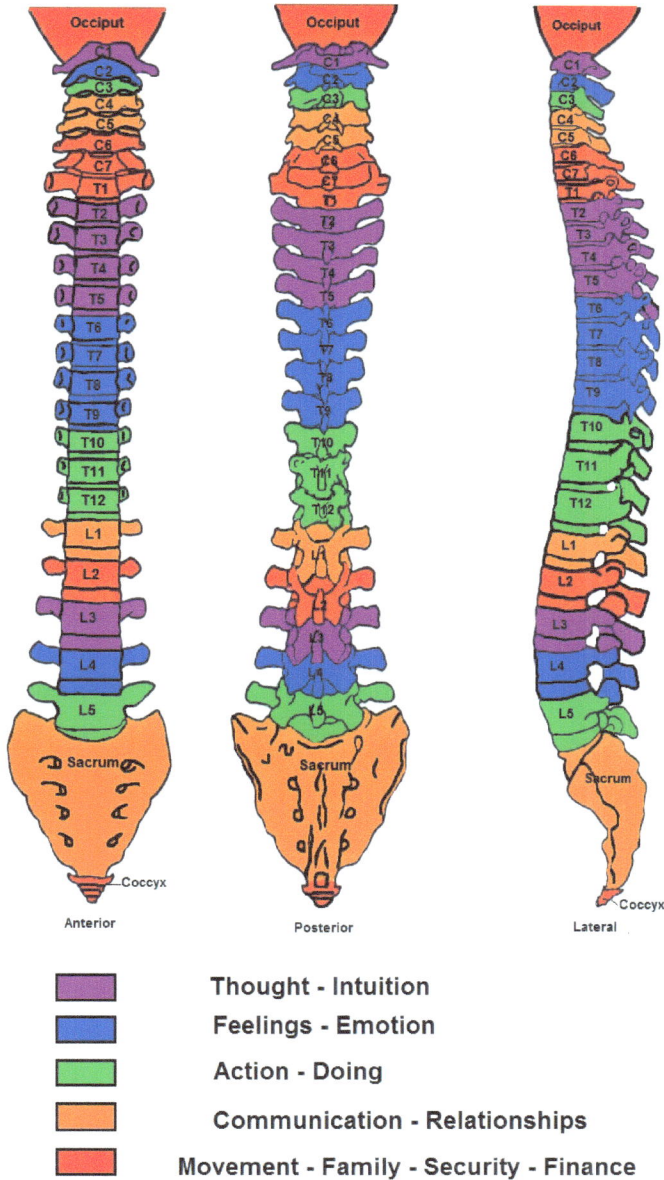

Thought - Intuition
Feelings - Emotion
Action - Doing
Communication - Relationships
Movement - Family - Security - Finance

Figure 1.9.4 Personality traits transposed to the spine (specific)

The following illustration (Figure 1.9.5) represents the product of the previous work. It describes how various negative emotions can affect the spine at various levels. It was presented on the Holistic Spine

115

poster and became the illustration that most practitioners made comment on, in that they perceived their various clients and patients in a new way. It goes without saying that I have also received negative comments from the scientific medical fraternity who insisted that I proved my findings in a scientific way.

Overall Picture   Detailed Picture

CRANIUM Insecurity, cannot earth or ground oneself

ATLAS Intuition, spirituality or intellect suppressed

AXIS Emotional imbalance, eye problems as child

C3 Pivot vertebra, undecided which way to turn

C4,5 Communication poor, cannot relate to others

C6, C7, T1 Worry over family, finance or security.

T2-T5 Suppressed thoughts of intuition causing asthma or chest tightness

T6-T9 Emotions dealing with the heart and love, also cowardice

T10-T12 How we assimilate things and move forward in our particular society

L1 Poor communicator, cannot form relationships

L2 Worries and stress with family and security

L3 Suppression of moving forward in life

L4 Emotional tension. Slighted by others as in bullying or divorce etc.

L5 Cannot move forward - stuck in a rut

Sacrum Tightens if cannot communicate. Relationships difficult

Coccyx Tense with fixed ideas in thoughts and ways

T Thought - Intuition

F Feelings - Emotion

A Action - Doing

C Communication - Relationships

M Movement - Family - Security - Finance

Once again, I shall not explain these findings in detail here as full explanations will be given as to the associations and reflections of each vertebral level in Part One of Book Two.

This completes Book One and I hope that you have enjoyed reading it. Book Two should be published in the early months of 2018. It will contain the following: -

BOOK TWO

Part One: Practical Considerations of each Vertebra

Each level of the spine will show the following associations and reflections – Spinal Nerve, Autonomic Nerve, Venous/Arterial, Major Chakra with Minor Chakra link, Acupuncture influence – Governor, Acupuncture influence – Bladder, Muscle tendon insertions, Linked Vertebra, Linked Organ, Mental and Spiritual.

Chapters

1. Sphenoid and Occiput

2. Atlas to C7

3. Thoracic Spine

4. Lumbar Spine

5. Sacrum, Coccyx and Sacroiliac joint

Part Two: Subtle Bodywork for Acute and Chronic Conditions

This section will discuss how to treat acute and chronic spinal conditions using various subtle bodywork techniques, acupressure and reflexology. This will include conditions associated with cranial nerves. The final chapter shows other miscellaneous attributes of the spine.

Chapters

6. Assessment
7. Sacro-Occipital therapy

8. Chinese Osteopathy in Cervical, Thoracic and Lumbo-Sacral conditions

9. Spinal Reflextherapy

10. Acupressure and Reflexology

11. Applied Kinesiology, Metamorphic Technique, Polarity Therapy, Colour and Sound Therapy in brief

References

Academy of Traditional Chinese Medicine. *An Outline of Chinese Acupuncture*. Beijing: Foreign Language Press, 1975

Brand, B. and Yancey P. *Fearfully and Wonderfully Made*. New York, USA: Zondervan Publishing, 1993

Cross, J.R. *Healing with the Chakra Energy System- Acupressure, Bodywork and Reflexology for Total Health*. Berkeley, California USA: North Atlantic Books, 2006

Cross, J.R. *Acupuncture and the Chakra Energy System – Treating the Cause of Disease*. Berkeley, California USA: North Atlantic Books, 2008

Cross, J.R. *The Concise Book of Acupoints*. Chichester UK: Lotus Publishing, 2010

Cross, J.R. *Reflected Energy Pathways – A Practical Workbook for Physical Therapists*. Chichester UK: Lotus Publishing, 2008

Gifford, Louis Ed. *Topical Issues in Pain 3 – Sympathetic Nervous System and Pain*. Physiotherapy Pain Association Bloomington, USA: Author House, 2013

Key, Sarah. *Sarah Key's Back Sufferers' Bible – You Can Treat Your Own Back*! London, UK: Random House, 2000

Lignon, Alain. *Schematisation Neuro-Vegetative En Osteopathie*. France: Editions de Verlaque, 2014 (In French)

Myers, T. *Anatomy Trains – Myofascial Meridians for Manual and Movement Therapists*. London and New York: Elsevier, 2014

Oliver, J and Middleditch, A. *Functional Anatomy of the Spine*. Oxford, UK: Butterworth-Heinemann, 1991

Sarno, J.E. *The Mind Body Prescription – Healing the Body, Healing the Pain*. New York, USA: Grand Central Lifestyle, 1998

Shapiro, D. *Your Body Speaks Your Mind – Understand How Your Thoughts and Emotions Affect Your Health*. London, UK. Piatkus, 1996

Stormer, C. *Language of the Feet – What Feet Can Tell You*. London, UK. Hodder and Stoughton, 1995

Williams, T. *Complete Chinese Medicine – A Comprehensive System for Health and Fitness*. Shaftesbury, Dorset UK. Element Books, 1996

I am indebted to the internet for several of the illustrations used in this book. With gratitude to Pinterest.

John Cross FCSP, Dr.Ac.
12 Upper Milovaig
Glendale
Isle of Skye
Highland
United Kingdom
IV55 8WY
Email - jrcacupressure@hotmail.com   or   johnc1112@yahoo.co.uk
Web site – www.johncrosspublications.com

www.ingramcontent.com/pod-product-compliance
Lightning Source LLC
Chambersburg PA
CBHW060804270326
41927CB00002B/43